Little Known Arthritis Treatments
Anthony di Fabio
Original Copyright January 10, 1995

Published by
The Arthritis Trust of America,
7111 Sweetgum Drive SW,
Fairview, TN 37062-9384
(615) 799-1002
Printed in USA

Dedication

Among those many open-minded physicians, scientists and new trend-setters who have helped shaped the content of this book are many giants. Chief among them, of course, are Professor Roger Wyburn-Mason, M.D., Ph.D., (deceased), Dr. Paul K. Pybus (deceased), Jack M. Blount, M.D., (deceased), Gus J. Prosch, Jr., M.D., (deceased) and Robert Bingham, M.D. (deceased). All were founders of The Arthritis Trust of America/The Rheumatoid Disease Foundation.

Whenever you find a physician who, like these giants, are sufficiently open-minded so as to work with you to explore and determine how to restore your health, and who are also willing to discard modalities which simply are not producing health, you've found a gem, a humanitarian, a physician of unimpeachable integrity. Stay with him/her!

So, along with the above mentioned men of great integrity, there were also nearly 200 physicians in 17 different countries (but mainly from the United States) of like mind on our Physician Referral List who have contributed to this book.

Chapter I
Introduction
Arthritis is incurable, you've been told!
Not so!
The vast majority of folks can and will get well if they will begin an active search for treatments that work. There are many treatments reported in this book that have been effective for tens of thousands.

If you have an interest in Arthritis, the chances are that you've been told that you have some form of Arthritis! Perhaps a doctor has heard your complaint, compared your symptoms against those that he knows, and then has named your "disease" with some sort of jawbreaker Latin.

The problem with labels -- as you and I know -- is that even if the one they've attached to your condition is the correct jawbreaker, knowing the disease's name does nothing by itself to relieve the pain or cure the condition. There is often a false presumption that knowing the name for a disease condition, or state of pain, leads to a correct remedy.

While it is sometimes true that naming a set of symptoms leads directly to an answer, such as in the use of antibiotics for sicknesses caused by known microorganisms, generally, and especially for debilitating diseases such as Arthritis, knowing the label is futile and can be misleading. Too often knowing the sophisticated jaw breaker medical term next leads to "Oh, that disease is not curable!"

Knowing the name of a disease state, and not knowing what to do about it to recover wellness, is frustration.

Two examples can be cited to demonstrate the limited usefulness and possible futility of classifying disease states when causation is unknown.

Prior to the discovery of the tubercle bacillus there were about 100 different names given to 100 different

4

presumed disease conditions. After the discovery of the tubercle bacillus, all of these 100 names collapsed into "tuberculosis of the bone," "of the skin," "of the lung," "of the spine," etc. In other words, the causation was the same, whereas the portion of the body affected, and showing symptoms, was different from person to person[1].

Medical history provides a second striking example in the nature of the symptoms of syphilis. If the syphilis spirochaete had not been discovered, the symptoms of syphilis would have fit a perfect example of proof of a defective immunological system -- exactly the situation that describes the predominant medical view of the causation of Rheumatoid Arthritis[1].

There are two acceptable explanations (or hypotheses) for describing the causation of Rheumatoid Arthritis. The predominant one is that something is akilter in the afflicted's immunological system. Why this possibility should lead to accepted drugs and treatments that further damage the immunological system appears to be an irrational medical act. Whereas, the other acceptable explanation -- that some unknown organism resides inside the afflicted's tissues, and the individual being genetically susceptible to either the organism or its toxins, reacts with an internal "allergic" reaction manifesting itself in the form of nearly 100 different named diseases -- does not lead to damaging drugs, and even points to successful therapies.

The Arthritis Trust of America/The Rheumatoid Disease Foundation takes the latter view, and now classifies the nearly 80 different disease states under the one heading of "Rheumatoid Diseases," or "Collagen Tissue Diseases."

Without a great deal of scientific and medical study it is futile to require a determination of which of the above two explanations is most probable. Probably both ideas have some truth, and, in fact, possibly many other factors are also related to a painful "arthritic" condition.

The human body, as with other mammals, operates by means of thousands, if not millions, of homeostatic systems. These are self-regulating mechanisms that operate to restore, within certain tolerances, a prior condition. Many years ago a Bell Laboratories speaker carried about a small black-box illustrating this principle. To open the box, one flipped an external toggle switch attached to the box. When the box was opened by human hand, a simulated human hand normally lying at rest inside the box activated, and before closing, the simulated human hand reached out of the box and flicked the external toggle switch causing the box to close again whence the simulated human hand recessed back into the box to rest again, just before the lid closed on it.

In like manner, whenever we affect a biological system, something natural to our organic mechanisms causes our automatic processes to restore to their initial or "home" status.

Some scientists and physicians view the disease or pain state as a mal-adaption condition, where our bodies, to function at all, must sustain an unnatural state which includes the pain that we subjectively sense. A crude example, using the black box with the internal simulated hand that restores homeostasis: suppose at the time the external toggle switch is triggered to open the box by a human hand, a stick is placed between the lid and the box. Then, the box's simulated human hand would reach out to trigger the external switch but could not reach it because the stick now interferes with completion of the action, and so the simulated human hand would in futility continue again and again trying to trigger the external switch. In the human body, the equivalent of trying to reach the toggle switch again and again, and failing, might be the human body's constant manufacture of a chemical designed to restore a prior condition which, because of our diet, or drugs, or environmental condition or some other unknown factors, prevents the chemicals from completing their function. The result, therefore, is a persistent attempt that fails, and possible pain.

We see this condition in Rheumatoid Diseases, where macrophages persistently attempt to kill organisms, and in so doing, also damage collagen tissue, which, in turn, creates secondary and tertiary damage to tissues and joints. However, it's overly simplistic to reason that the "cause" of the disease is the macrophage, implying that the afflicted have an improper immunological system. This over-simplistic explanation leads to ways and means to further damage the macrophages at the expense of the whole immunological system, and consequently the whole human body. This additional damage then creates more of the equivalent of probing hands failing in attempts to turn off more toggle switches, thereby creating more maladaptations.

It is rare, in the annals of medicine, that a single cause of a disease state can be known, and, if known, can be treated as distinct from all other physiological relationships.

It is more usual, especially with Arthritides (Arthritides: a collective term applied to various joint disorders) that multiple-causations are suspect, and that multiple treatments be simultaneously used to restore a better quality of life.

More than likely you're reading this book because you've tried established medical procedures, and failed to relieve your problem.

You also hope that our suggestions will bear fruit, and are worthy of the expense often required to get well.

The Arthritis Arthritis Trust of America/The Rheumatoid Disease Foundation has since 1982 generously helped folks to get well by finding for them knowledgeable physicians and recommending appropriate treatments. Success rate has been high for those afflicted who are willing to begin the grand search of "learning what works for me."

Early statistics kept by our referral physicians demonstrated that 80% of those who followed our recommendations got well from crippling Rheumatoid Diseases, providing they hadn't already been treated by traditional means of long-term corticosteroids, gold shots, penicillamine or methotrexate, or other cytotoxic drugs. If they have been so abused by these damaging treatments, affecting the ability of their biology to respond, our treatment recommendation's percentage of successes dropped to 50%, which is still considerably greater than the "improvement" rate of about 33% obtained through the traditional treatments.

Incidently, that 33% "improvement" rate claimed by established treatments is just about equal to the placebo effect. That is, about 33% of the afflicted will "improve," from time to time, no matter what, within limits, is done to them[1,11].

There are many kinds of Arthritides determined by observation of symptoms, each named uniquely. The three most prominent are Osteoarthritis, Rheumatoid Arthritis and Gouty Arthritis. There are also many pains and other symptoms that resemble, or mimic, some of the above. In the process of untangling one thing from another, and taking over the responsibility for your own wellness, you'll learn, or must learn, to fix what's wrong with you.

Chapter II
Painful "Arthritis"

Pain and joint dysfunction may derive from certain not-well-known physiological maladaptations, or may result as a matter of processes that mimic these maladaptations.

There are many kinds of arthritides. The most common are three: Osteoarthritis, Rheumatoid Arthritis and Gouty Arthritis. The causation of those that may mimic any of these, or combinations of these, may derive from allergies, effects of pollutants, chemical imbalances, Candidiasis and other microorganisms, dental mercury and other metal toxicities, physical sports accidents and so on.

Tens of millions of Americans suffer from either Osteo Arthritis or Gouty Arthritis, while at least thirteen million Americans suffer from improperly classified "incurable" Rheumatoid Disease, a name given to a broad cluster of diseases, perhaps 80 in number, that, while appearing to be different diseases because they are described by different word-labels, are nonetheless all related by the fact that collagen tissue is somehow affected.

An estimated forty million people have Osteoarthritis, six million have Rheumatoid Arthritis and about one million Americans have Gouty Arthritis[1,2,3,4,5]

Most people know "arthritis" as a joint disease: painful, swollen or heated joints. Most treatments, therefore, are aimed at relieving pain at the joints without in any way attending to the "systemic" nature of the diseases. "Systemic" means that the disease is pervasive, throughout the whole body.

It has been stated by some practicing physicians that at least 50% of us will have Osteoarthritis (Osteo) if we live long enough, and therefore Osteoarthritis is often -- probably wrongly -- said to be a "degenerative" or "aging" disease. It is characterized by swelling that is bony with irregular spurs and occasional soft cysts, whereas Rheumatoid Arthritis is characterized by synovial, capsular soft tissue that is bony only in late stages[3].

Tenderness is normal for Rheumatoid Arthritis, but is

usually absent with Osteoarthritis, except during occasional acute flare-ups and particularly at the onset. The distal interphalangeal joint (closest to the nails) is usually not involved with Rheumatoid Arthritis (except thumb) but quite characteristic with Osteo. The proximal interphalangeal joint (middle) is usually involved with Rheumatoid Arthritis, and is frequently involved with Osteo. The metacarpophalangeal joint (knuckles) is usually involved with Rheumatoid Arthritis, but never with Osteo, except for the thumb. Wrist involvement is normal for Rheumatoid Arthritis but never involved with Osteo, except for the base of the thumb[3].

Osteoarthritis is characterized by degenerative loss of joint cartilage, deadening of bone beneath the cartilage, and cartilage and bone proliferation at the joint margins with subsequent bony outgrowths. Impaired joint function and synovial inflammation is common[3].

Osteoarthritis is said to be "inflammation of the bones and joints" according to a medical dictionary.

While Osteo is painful, and leads to progressively less usage of joints, it is not the great crippler that characterizes Rheumatoid Arthritis. Rheumatoid Arthritis usually is known by a cluster of easily observed symptoms distinguishing it from Osteo: Joints are swollen, heated, and an increasing number of them become affected over time. Night sweats, depression and lethargy accompany this disease[1].

Gouty Arthritis, on the other hand, is characterized by sharp painful joints, as if a needle were probing the internal structure of the joints. One can have attacks of fever, chills and, of course, the described excruciating needlelike pains. Gout victims will suffer for weeks at a time often with loss of mobility; and, as these attacks become more frequent, they will eventually be disabling. Kidney disease, heart disease, and many other complications can set in[5].

Chapter III
Osteoarthritis
What Causes Osteoarthritis?

Osteoarthritis appears to be caused by a combination of factors. Hormonal deficiencies certainly play their part, as one-third more women suffer from Osteoarthritis after menopause than do men. Faulty nutrition and stress may also play their fair share, as probably do genetic predisposing factors[1,2,3,4].

Prevailing general medical theory suggests that Osteoarthritis may be divided into two categories, primary and secondary[17]. "In primary osteoarthritis, the degenerative `wear-and-tear' process occurs after the fifth and sixth decades, with no apparent predisposing abnormalities. The cumulative effects of decades of use leads to the degenerative changes by stressing the collagen matrix of the cartilage. Damage to the cartilage results in the release of enzymes that destroy collagen components. With aging, the ability to restore and synthesize normal collagen structures is decreased.

"Secondary osteoarthritis is associated with some predisposing factor which is responsible for the degenerative changes. Predisposing factors in secondary osteoarthritis include: congenital abnormalities in joint structure or function (e.g., hypermobility and abnormally shaped joint surfaces); trauma (obesity, fractures along joint surfaces, surgery, etc.); crystal deposition; presence of abnormal cartilage; and previous inflammatory disease of joint (rheumatoid arthritis, gout, septic arthritis, etc.)[3,4]"

Prevention Of Osteoarthritis

There are, apparently, three major aspects to the prevention of Osteoarthritis: restore proper nutrition, relieve stress and replace hormones[3,4].

Nutrition must be designed to fit each individual, of

course, but there are always good broad outlines that are safe and helpful for each of us. According to Gus J. Prosch, Jr. M.D.[95], in principle the closer we can eat to the "caveman diet" the better the nutritional values received. Our human bodies evolved through a varying diet of grains, nuts, berries, fish, meats and other food substances. The "caveman diet" is generally described by recommendations of <u>fresh</u> fruits and vegetables, whole grains, nuts, cold water fish and other sources of essential fatty acids.

One mineral apparently of great importance to the prevention of Osteoarthritis is boron. Dr. Rex E. Newnham, Ph.D., D.O., N.D. of Leeds, England demonstrated demographic and clinical evidence for the usefulness of Boron in preventing and treating Osteoarthritis and some forms of Rheumatoid Disease[3,4]. Fluoridated water, besides contributing to Osteoporosis, and other degenerative diseases, including Skeletal Fluorosis, which many doctors call "Arthritis," without in any way helping the teeth or bones, also is a natural antagonist to boron, and so Dr. Newnham recommends removing the Fluoride from your water if you are to get benefit from Boron. Furthermore, if you make tea with fluoridated water, there is much more fluoride in your tea than the cold water alone. For Arthritis, Rheumatism and Osteoporosis, he recommends the use of tablets containing Boron (Sodium Tetraborate) 2.6 mg, Calcium Ascorbate 200 mg, Magnesium Ascorbate 90 mg, Pyridoxine 2.6 mg, Zinc (as Citrate) 4.5 mg, Manganese (as Citrate) 4.5 mg, Copper (as Citrate) .46 mg, Nicotinamide 10 mg, Herbs 10 mg. Such a mixture he has patented under the name of Osteo Trace[TM]. Dr. Newnham recommends 3 tablets a day, one with each meal, if under 168 pounds, 4 tablets a day if over 168 pounds but under 210 pounds, and 5 tablets a day if over 210 pounds. Children between 50 and 100 pounds weight, 2 tablets per day, and infants under 20 pounds only half a tablet per day[110].

William Kaufman, Ph.D., M.D.[89,90,91] demonstrated over many years of clinical practice the reversal of Osteoarthritis and some Rheumatoid Disease dysfunction by use of Niacinamide together with other vitamins and minerals.

Dietary supplements often used are: Niacinamide[89,90,91] (under close medical supervision), Methionine, Glycosaminoglycans, Superoxide Dismutase, Vitamins A, E, Pyridoxine, Pantothenic Acid and minerals Zinc and Copper[18].

Linus Pauling Ph.D.[64] and Robert F. Cathcart, III M.D.[2] both recommend large quantities of Vitamin C, either orally or as an injectable.

Many of the above supplements are antioxidants, anti-inflammatories, synergistic with other substances, hormonal replacements or blockages, or intended to encourage the maintenance of, or faster regrowth of, connective tissue.

Various herbs[60] have been historically useful for the same purposes, especially in treating inflammation without the serious side-affects attributed to aspirin and other Non-Steroidal Anti-Inflammatories (NSAIDS). These are *Glycyrrhiza glabra*, *Medicago sativa*, *Harpagophytum procumbens*, and the Proanthocyanidins, Cherries, Hawthorn Berries and Blueberries[17,19].

Stress[69] is a factor that is perhaps most often overlooked by the normal medical practitioner. Often there is one or more persons in the close work or home environment who are suppressive to another, such suppression expressing itself in a way that constantly invalidates a person's actions, thoughts or emotions. It is a negative stimulus that depresses our beingness, our will to want to engage in friendly exchange of ideas or activities. A person who is so related to another will often suppress his/her emotions and behavior in ways that express outwardly in the form of hormonal changes and accompanying clinical sicknesses. The medical terminology is "psychosomatic," indicating that the person's mind governs his emotions and bodily condition. This is true to the extent that a person permits suppressive conditions and "suppressive" people to influence his/her mind/body. As few physicians have training in recognizing the causative patterns, and would probably be resisted by their patients if they mentioned them, stress sources are often ignored in treatment, although they may be the largest component of all diseases, acute or chronic[2,12].

Hormonal replacement therapy is practiced by many physicians who recognize that our organs decrease in ability to perform as we age. Their goal is to achieve a natural balance of all hormonal factors, which is presumed to be an assist to restoration of health that was once ours. The fact that Osteoarthritis is most frequent among women after menopause is a critical clue, as both estrogen and progesterone may be decreased or unbalanced with aging and especially after menopause. According to Raymond F. Peat, Ph.D., "Stress-induced cortisone deficiency is thought to be a factor in a great variety of unpleasant conditions, from allergies to ulcerative colitis, and in some forms of arthritis. The stress which can cause a cortisone deficiency is even more likely to disturb formation of progesterone and thyroid hormone, so the fact that cortisone can relieve symptoms does not mean that it has corrected the problem.

"Besides the thyroid, the other class of adaptive hormones which are often out of balance in the diseases of stress, is the group of hormones produced mainly by the gonads: the 'reproductive hormones'.[73]" There is often need to consider hormonal replacement, not just in serious cases of thyroid deficiency, but also in marginal cases. A physician who understands the relationship between stress, hormones and disease should be consulted, and, in the case of determining Thyroid deficiency borderline cases, many will recommend the method of Broda Barnes, M.D.[6,33] who developed a method based on taking armpit temperature before arising every morning, as laboratory testing is not geared to discover marginal deficiencies[6].

Dehydroepiandrosterone (DHEA) may also be an important and relevant replacement hormone, as described in the Rheumatoid Disease section that follows[96].

Treatment Of Osteoarthritis

Treatment for Osteoarthritis -- or what appears to be Osteoarthritis -- can be divided into four components: Treatment for the (1) pain, (2) defective skeletal structure, (3) faulty nutrition, (4) hormonal imbalances.

As treatment for faulty nutrition and hormonal imbalances has already been mentioned, and as they both require individualized attention by holistically minded physicians, we shall further discuss only treatment for pain and defective skeletal structure, with the exception of repeated emphasis on the use of niacinamide as per William Kaufman's Ph.D. M.D. early and lengthy research work[89,90,91].

Pain and Defective Structure

Professor Roger Wyburn-Mason M.D, Ph.D. more than thirty-five years ago was able to demonstrate that the source of pain in both Osteoarthritis and Rheumatoid Disease is not in the joints — where most modern-day treatment lies — but in certain key nerve ganglia leading to the joint. These nerve ganglia are found in uninsulated nerves usually lying close to the skin's surface, known as "C fibers."

Intra-Neural Injections

Based on Roger Wyburn-Mason's theory, Dr. Paul Pybus[7] found that a combination of Depot Medrol with a very dilute solution of Triamcinolone Hexacetonide (Lederspan® or Aristospan®) not only immediately halted the pain appearing in remote joints, but also permitted the nerve cell lesions to heal, probably by stabilizing nerve cell membranes.

Pybus stated that these nerve lesions triggered off two signals, one set following the nerve path to the brain, the other following a reflex arc to the spinal column and back. The signal to the brain came back to represent pain at the joint. The reflex signal to the spinal column came back to the joint to produce the following easily recognizable phenomena: heated joints (pyrexia), swollen joints (edema) and tension or clamping of muscles at the joints. **It is the tension or clamping of muscles at the joints which creates degeneration of cartilage at the joint which results in the pain of Osteoarthritis (or the pain of Rheumatoid Arthritis),** and this was further explained by Pybus by knowledge of Charnley clamps used on knee joints which, while producing a forcible compression of joints, also resulted in destruction of cartilage in the joints.

Destruction of cartilage (leading to pyrexia and edema) is caused because cartilage, having virtually no blood distribution system of its own, requires a continuous squeezing and expanding of the cartilage in the joint, squeezing out blood and sponging it up, respectively. When joints are under conscious or unconscious tension because of nerve cell lesions constantly sending a reflex signal to tense or clamp the joint — then the cartilage begins to degenerate through lack of sufficient nourishment and this decomposition results in the creation of additional secondary and tertiary "free radical" chemical reactions that are further destructive, also producing the symptoms of pyrexia (heat) and edema (swelling). "Free radicals" are chemicals that seek active combination with other chemicals.

Gus J. Prosch, Jr., M.D.[95] successfully developed the Wyburn-Mason/Pybus intraneural treatment for arthritics in the United States, and taught many physicians.

Acupuncture

Most of the traditional acupuncture points are exactly the same as the trigger or key nerve ganglia used in Intraneural Injections, and the physics of explanation is identical for both, as the developer of Intraneural Injections, Dr. Paul Pybus, was first an acupuncturist and then a surgeon. He said, "Acupuncture . . . shows no great permanency in the relief afforded just by one treatment, as when the needle is removed the membrane is still destabilized and the condition reverts to the status quo ante." This seems to be confirmed by the experience of Arabinda Das, M.D. who says, "acupuncture may help localized pain of rheumatoid arthritis but chronic generalized rheumatoid arthritis is not amenable to acupuncture as [is true with] many chronic infectious conditions[79]."

When Pybus combined acupuncture with a substance that stabilized the nerve cell membrane, he began to see long-term improvement in both Osteoarthritis and the pain of Rheumatoid Arthritis. Undoubtedly others who were familiar with Acupuncture discovered this same phenomenon, as there is now practiced "Pharmaceutical Acupuncture."

In addition to good effects on pain, Acupuncture is said to strengthen the immune system[69].

Electromagnetics and Biomagnetics

In the past practice of medicine chemistry has been applied to the human body more than the knowledge of physics. Many physicians and researchers are now exploring physics in relation to the body, and one important area is the effect of electromagnetics and/or powerful specially built (i.e. ceramic) magnetics primarily for the relief of pain[53,112]."

As the use of magnets, and their accompanying magnetic fields, interfere with the natural magnetic field of the cells and the body, one must be very careful not to use these magnetics indiscriminately.

There is often confusion between the use of electromagnetics and magnetics, and there are reports of serious damage having been done to individuals who have used magnetics of powerful force, thus having interfered with the body's natural fields. Thus, ELF Laboratories[113,114,115,116], and others caution against the use of magnetics, but do recommend the use of pulsating electromagnetic fields under certain very carefully controlled conditions. One such condition is the combination use of the Light Beam Generator with the Vodder Lymphatics Massage technique assisted by a flow of harmless electrons, that has beneficial effects on the body's cells.

This is described in a later section.

Niacinamide and Boron

The excellent work of Dr. Rex Newnham, Ph.D., D.O., N.D. has already been mentioned with regard to Boron. Through demographic analysis, and later clinical trials, he was able to demonstrate that both Osteoarthritis and Rheumatoid Disease can be stemmed through appropriate quantities of Boron[23].

Also of special importance is the excellent work of William Kaufman, M.D., Ph.D. in the use of Niacinamide for both Osteoarthritis and Rheumatoid Arthritis. Dr. Kaufman, through clinical observation, determined that Aniacinamidosis (lack of sufficient niacinamide) was persistent with those having joint problems of Osteoarthritis or Rheumatoid Arthritis. He invented a measuring device easy for other doctors to use, and thus standardized by an objective measure improvement, or lack of, in patients. Over many years and with the help of many patients, including those with aging problems, Dr. Kaufman developed an oral schedule of niacinamide per day, the Niacinamide being taken in frequent intervals during the day in, usually, varying dosages because of the quickness by which niacinamide flushed from the body[89,90,91]. Usually the dosage is dependent upon severity of the joint dysfunction.

Neural And Reconstructive Therapy

Another cause of the pain of Osteoarthritis is defective skeletal posture resulting in pains remote from the source of defect or misalignment, and also pain from Osteoarthritic calcium spurs usually located along the spinal column and rubbing on branching nerves from the spine[8]. Possibly the first treatment of choice by Osteoarthritics should be that known by D.O.'s as "Sclerotherapy", by M.D's. as "Proliferative Therapy", and by some modern-day physicians as "Reconstructive Therapy".

Strangely enough, and little known by many physicians, scar tissue from past penetrations of the skin can also cause skeletal misalignment problems, and these are usually treated at the same time using Neural/ FascialTherapy[9], a treatment developed by German physicians, and especially Ferdinand Huenke, M.D. and Walter Huenke, M.D.[16]. The knowledgeable patient will find a physician who practices these two treatment modalities before trying many other forms of treatment.

More than 30 years ago demonstrations on laboratory animals showed that loosened, stretched or torn tendons and ligaments could be tightened up by means of inserting just beneath the skin, in the proper location, a natural bodily substance (Sodium Morrhuate) which would promote the growth of collagen tissue and fibroblasts. Other substances besides Sodium Morrhuate are also used.

As we age, our tendons and ligaments tend to stretch or can be torn from their connections to fascia through sports or accidents, or can be weakened through poor nutrition, disease or unbalanced chemistries. As the body's skeletal posture is held together by means of tendons and ligaments — not the muscles per se — a stretching of one set of tendons or ligaments will be unconsciously compensated for by other pulley and lever mechanisms in remote parts of the body. According to masseur Thomas Gervais[88], "Tendons are muscle ends. Fascia apparently gives ligaments and bones their proper place/structure. The fascial connective tissue thickens and becomes most rigid at places of greatest/most frequent use and demand. This `ossification' process of fascia makes a return to good posture difficult." One compensatory mechanism is the production of Osteoarthritic spurs in the spine. Although the body's problem is lax or torn ligaments or tendons elsewhere, the body's chemistry attempts to compensate by creating calcium spurs along the spinal column. Were these calcium spurs cut out, the body's tendon and/or ligament problems would persist, and the body would attempt to compensate in additional ways.

To illustrate: James A. Carlson, D.O. was asked to look at a patient's right index finger-joint nearest to the fingernail (between the Distal phalanx and the Middle phalanx). The joint had been inflamed for months and was deforming. After study Dr. Carlson deduced that the cause was a left-foot heel-bone out of alignment. This may sound peculiar until one is versed with the manner in which the skeleton is held together, and the means by which the human body compensates. A bone awry at one

place affects structure remotely connected. Using Osteo-
pathic manipulation, he placed the heel bone back, and
then using reconstructive therapy, Dr. Carlson placed near
the proper tendons and ligaments substances that promote
the body's ability to keep the bone in place. The finger
immediately ceased its pain and deformation stopped[10].

In a similar instance, the finger nearest the small one
on the left hand was unable to touch the palm of the hand.
It was very stiff and often hurt. Dr. Carlson determined that
the cause was an arch-bone in the left foot out of alignment. Again he manipulated the bone to its proper location
and then used reconstructive therapy to place the bone
permanently where it belonged. The pain immediately
disappeared and the patient had restored ability to touch
the palm of the hand with that finger[10].

Many other instances -- much more spectacular[8,9] -
- can be described for all parts of the body where
Osteoarthritis is presumed but in fact it is the slackness or
disruption at the connective base of ligaments and tendons
that slowly create Osteoarthritic-like symptoms[8].

According to William Faber, D.O. and Morton Walker,
D.P.M., "typical musculoskeletal lesions that may be
permanently corrected are: bunions, heel difficulties, finger dysfunctions, patellar problems, migraine headache,
neck pain, chronic shoulder dislocation, rotator cuff tears,
generalized back weakness, herniated disks, mid-level
backache, low back pain, compression fractures of the
vertebrae, ankylosing spondylitis, spondylolisthesis, fi-
brositis, fascitis, tendonitis, pain after severe injury, pain
after stroke, temporomandibular joint (TMJ) syndrome,
post-orthopedic surgery pain, dysfunctional hip joint,
chronic and acute knee disability, ankle weakness, tennis
leg, tennis elbow, wrist pain, carpal-tunnel syndrome, and
most forms of arthritis, especially the type derived from
wear and tear (osteoarthritis), and more disabilities. Re-

constructive therapy is often a medical alternative to orthopedic surgery, hand surgery, podiatric surgery and other traditional techniques of musculoskeletal repair[8]."

According to Gus Prosch, Jr., M.D., Intraneural Injections and Reconstructive Therapy cannot be performed at the same time, as the chemistry of the two therapies work in opposition to one another[2,8].

Rolfing®

To solve what was diagnosed as Rheumatoid Disease, Ida P. Rolf, Ph.D.[86] developed and applied her "massage" discovery in what is now called "Rolfing"[2]. Dr. Rolf may or may not have had Rheumatoid Disease, but her discovery has wide application to all forms of arthritides, as well as other structural and pain problems.

According to the Rolf Institute[87], founded to carry on Dr. Rolf's work, "Fascia belongs to a family of closely related connective tissues found throughout the human body. Although fascia is technically a tissue, Rolfers sometimes speak of it as the `organ of form' because it literally holds your body together and gives it shape." Fascia is found throughout the body and surrounds all organs. If healthy, it is slightly elastic with strong resistance to stretching. It can break or tear however.

The nature of fascia is to fasten and hold. According to the Rolf Institute: "1) Slack strands of fascia can adhere to one another [adhesions] and shorten a fascial structure, thus distorting the three-dimensional fascial network and pulling the skeleton (and body segments) out of alignment. This can occur in response to poor postural or movement patterns, injury, [chronic emotional patterns] or surgery. . . .) Adjacent fascial structures can adhere to one another and bind two structures together. Even in a healthy body, the fascial envelopes of adjacent muscles may adhere to one another. Two muscles, which should glide over each other, become yoked together; neither muscle can function independently and efficiently."

Fascia can adhere to itself and change shape causing the fascial network to become distorted, but this plasticity, fortunately, can also work in the other direction, restoring the structural integrity with the proper Rolfing applications of pressure.

According to Dr. Ida Rolf, ". . . the `joint' is much more than the bone of the ball-and-socket. All muscles and ligaments that weave or support its structure are part of it. This is true of any joint. Trouble in any of the component parts -- muscles, ligaments, bones -- is apt to be interpreted or at least verbalized as being in the joint. Unnumbered, casual, hasty diagnoses of `arthritis' reflect nothing more serious than a shortened or displaced muscle or ligament resulting from a recent or not-so-recent traumatic episode. True arthritis, on the other hand, is deterioration of the joint, characterized by chemical change in the blood and in joint tissue. Arthritic pain is the result of joint compression. Not all cases of true arthritis are painful; where there is adequate capsular space, the individual may well be pain-free. When your shoulder or your hip hurts, it is well to paraphrase an old adage: not only is all that glitters not gold, but, even more hopeful, all that hurts is not necessarily arthritis. It may be merely pseudoarthritis, a disorder in the tendons and ligaments. . . . Appropriate muscular organization can give the pseudoarthritic movements and render him pain-free."

Rolfing, through restoration of fascial integrity, restores natural posture which, for the arthritic and pseudoarthritic alike, means more freedom of movement and lessened pain, and also improvement of metabolism, circulation, neural transmission, joint and tissue repair, emotional stability, and, generally, an overall increase in available energy that was otherwise bound up in maintaining the poor muscular imbalances.

Other Treatments
Photopheresis
Photopheresis is a new form of treatment that exposes portions of the blood mixed with a light-sensitive chemical to ultraviolet radiation. Its object is to "immunize" the body against malignant T cells found in the immunological system. It has so far shown promise for the treatment of various Rheumatoid Diseases (Scleroderma, Lupus Erythematosus, Rheumatoid Arthritis), autoimmune diabetes mellitus, organ transplant rejection and AIDS related complex[25]. William Campbell Douglass, M.D. of Georgia reports excellent success with many otherwise intransigent disease conditions, using photopheresis, and especially against AIDS[26].

Cryogenic Exposure and Exercise Treatment
Japanese scientists demonstrated the improved effects of cryogenic exposure on degenerative disease. Tonis Pai[27], M.D. of Tallin, Estonia, who constructed his own clinic's cryogenic chamber, also continues this work reporting improvement among patients with various joint diseases, including Rheumatoid Arthritis and Osteoarthritis. Patients enter a chamber (cooled cryogenically by liquid nitrogen) for repeated visits for a duration of 1-3 minutes. They then exercise strenuously.

Ge-132: Bis-Beta-carboxyethyl: Germanium Sesquioxide
Dr. K. Asai of Japan designed Bis-Beta-carboxyethyl Germanium Sesquioxide (Ge-132), finding thereafter many interesting and useful properties. Ge-132 is a substance that does not easily enter into bodily tissues, and therefore has been found to be non-dangerous. It performs several valuable functions, among which is the ability to take up excess electrons from the cell's mitochondria -- the cell's power unit -- and flush them from the body. This function is analogous to increasing basal metabolism at the cellular

24

level. Excess electrons can create free-radicals which may lead to pain and inflammation. Ge-132 also decreases pain by increasing endorphins in the brain. "In both humans and animals Ge-132 has been shown to increase gamma interferon in the blood, activate macrophages and natural killer cells, bring blood hemoglobin levels up and white cell counts down, stimulate immunomodulation activity in the B cell system and demonstrate antitumor and antiviral activities. This substance, therefore, may be an excellent adjuvant (aids the operation) of immunochemotherapeutic agents. The effects of Ge-132 on various immune parameters are almost identical to that of known gamma interferon immunomodulating activity. In addition, studies on immune-suppressed animals and on patients with malignancies or rheumatoid arthritis suggest that Ge-132 normalized the function of T cells, B lymphocytes, antibody-dependent cellular cytotoxicity, natural killer cell activity and numbers of antibody-forming cells. Obviously organic germanium has a `normalizing' influence on the immune system[57,58,59]," and it can be effectively used either sub-lingually or as an injectable.

Caution: do not take Germanium Oxide, which is poisonous and can be damaging.

Live-Cell Therapy

According to Lester Winters, Ph.D.[93,100], and Robert Bradford, D.Sc.[111], European Live-Cell Therapy has been available for many years, and used by millions of people. Prof. Paul Niehans, a famous Swiss physician and Surgeon, is considered the father of cellular therapy used by kings and queens, popes, presidents, ministers, movie stars and the wealthy. Pioneer Wolfram Kuhnau, M.D. reported that past recipients of Live-Cell Therapy included "Konrad Adenauer, Charles DeGaulle, Dwight D. Eisenhower, Sir Winston Churchill, the Duke and Duchess of Windsor, Haile Selassi, the monarchs of Moracco and Saudi Arabia, Bernard Baruch, and Joseph Kennedy[110]." This replacement therapy now is available at a reasonable cost outside of the United States in Europe, Bahamas, Mexico and other countries. Briefly, calf, sheep or piglet fetal (embryonic) tissue is injected (or placed) in the body. (Apparently any mammalian tissue will do, so long as it is from the proper fetal stage, kept sterile, and stored properly, although bovine or sheep tissues, for various reasons, are preferred by many.) For a period of one to four years, depending upon nutrition, metabolism and life-style, these foreign tissues supply hormones and other vital chemicals which the body uses as its own. Of greater significance, is the ability of the body to repair damaged molecules in fading organs, thus restoring vitality and health. Additionally, according to Dr. med. Gerhard Shettler[94], intra-articular cellular therapy is often effective in replacing damaged or worn joint cartilage. William Saccoman, M.D. has had considerable success replacing joint cartilage[100].

Live-cell therapy is well worth trying for various health reasons, not just Osteoarthritis and Rheumatoid Diseases. A listing, according to Bradford[110], follows: "Neuromuscular disorders, including epilepsy, multiple sclerosis, amytrophic lateral sclerosis (ALS), Parkinson's, post-stroke paralysis and muscular dystrophy; hormone-dependent dysfunctions including a full range of sexual disorders ranging from impotence and early menopause as well as obesity, insufficiency and hypothyroidism; chronic dermatological disorders, especially psoriasis and eczema; chronic arthritis of all kinds; chronic pancreatitis; arteriosclerosis; liver cirrhosis; allergies of all kinds; genetic and hereditary disorders, including mental retardation, Down's syndrome, bone and cartilage abnormalities, congenital hip malformations, congenital dysplasias, spinal problems, cleft lip and palate; chronic lung disease;

chronic kidney disease; autoimmune disease; narcolepsy; and rejuvenation[111]."

The arthritides afflicted would do well to explore this approach.

Homeopathy

Homeopathy is several centuries old, and was once a widely practiced healing discipline, until the dominance of allopathic medicine in many parts of the world. Allopathy, the dominant medical philosophy in the United States, is that method which seeks to cure disease by the production of a condition of the system either different from or opposite to the condition produced by the disease[101]. Homeopathy is its opposite, a theory or system of curing diseases with very minute doses of medicine which in a healthy person and in large doses would produce a condition like that of the disease treated[101]. The basic principle is that symptoms of a "disease" are a natural part of the healing process. As such, they must be allowed to occur, even augmented, rather than be suppressed.

According to the Arizona Revised Statutes 32-2901, "Homeopathy means a system of medicine employing substances of animal, vegetable or mineral origin which are given in microdosage, prepared according to homeopathic pharmacology, in accordance with the principle that a substance which produces symptoms in a healthy person can cure those symptoms in an ill person. The practice of homeopathy [in Arizona] includes acupuncture, neuromuscular integration, orthomolecular therapy, nutrition, chelation therapy, pharamaceutical medicine and minor surgery[66]." As some practitioners of Homeopathy do not subscribe to the total practice as described herein, we will discuss only the first part of the above definition.

Dr. Samuel Hahneman (one of Napoleon Bonaparte's physicians[66,69]), Kent[66], and others founded and defined the basic outlines of Homeopathy. On Napoleon's route to conquer most of Europe, Napoleon used "Dr. Hahneman to keep his troops free of typhoid fever. Hahneman created a totally new concept of medicine, which he called `Homeopathy,' derived from the Greek words, `homeos,' which means `similar,' and, `pathos' or `disease'. Hahneman's basic law was, `Let's cure a disease with the disease itself, or like cures like[69]." Hahneman and other physicians observed and reported that an extremely minute dosage of a substance that could reproduce some of the symptoms of a known disease could somehow teach the body how to heal itself. Substances, therefore, are diluted to such an extreme dilution that scoffing scientists will describe the resulting mixture as being the "essence of residual vibrations of a ghostly spirit passing quickly through the room one time."

Carefully selected substances are sequentially diluted (and struck: percussed) to concentrations such as 0.9×10^{-61}. The more diluted is the substance chosen, the more "powerful" its effect -- a phenomenon which stretches normal imagination beyond training of allopathic physicians.

While it is true that modern medicine has a difficult time reconciling healing with a dilution so tiny that no molecule of the original substance can possibly remain, there are efforts to develop hypotheses to explain the mystery. Several clinical experiments have stood up to scrutiny, including increase in growth of wheat seedlings, diastase hydrolysis of starch and lymphoblast growth rate. Studies using nuclear magnetic resonance spectra, photoelectric densities and dielectric constants have been made, and new hypotheses have been created, seeking a "rational" explanation[67]. To the great chagrin and consternation of traditional allopathic practitioners, "*The British Medical Journal* (Feb. 9, 1991) published a groundbreaking survey of clinical research on homeopathic medicine. Three experts on clinical research analyzed 107 controlled clinical studies which were published between 1966 and 1990. They noted that 81 trials indicated positive results[70]."

While Homeopathy is not licensed in all states, it has been available in many European countries for 200 years. Certain present-day royalty and other governmental leaders would not have any other kind. And, while John D. Rockerfeller (the original) is said to have promoted allopathy in many American medical schools -- as drugs increased his profits -- he, himself, would not permit any other kind of physician than one who practiced Homeopathy.

In addition to healing, Homeopathy is said to strengthen the immune system[69]. Many success stories, with every form of disease, have been reported through the use of Homeopathy. According to Corazon Ilarina, M.D.[40], recommended Homeopathic remedies are Traumeel, Belladonna, Injul Farte arsemium, Album Injul, Hepeel, Injul-Chal, Phosphor Injul and Lachesis. She says that "Traumeel and Zeel ointments are very good for swelling and inflammation when applied topically on affected joints[40]." Dr. Ilarina also uses Homotoxicology which is the Homeopathic process of ridding the body of toxins that contribute to disease.

Recently, there has come increasing successes combining Homeopathy with work originally defined by Louis Pasteur's contemporary Antoine Bechamp. "Professor Dr. Guenther Enderlein (1872-1968) and his associate Alfred Baum, M.D. along with discoveries of German doctor Alexander von Seld, M.D. and Wilhelm von Brehmer[68]" state that they have developed Homeopathic medicines that cause pleomorphic organisms in one state to revert to a state capable of living amicably with the body, and they include a very wide range of diseases, including various arthritides, in their successes. (Also Ernst B. Almquist[77], Gerald J. Domingue[107], F.E. Haag[77], Koch[77], G. Koraen[77], Virginia Livingston-Wheeler, M.D.[83], A. Maffucci[77], Lida Mattman, Ph.D.[77], Gaston Naessen[84], P.G. Olsson[77], Royal Rife, E.J. Roukavischnikoff[77], Jorgan U. Schlegel, Gerda Troili-Petersson[77], Willibald Winkler, M.D.[77], Hannah B. Woody[78], W. Zopf[77], and many others[77], have followed up wholly or in part, or rediscovered, Antoine Bechamp's[76] work but applied concepts not necessarily related to Homeopathy.)

Dehydroepiandrosterone (DHEA Sulfate) Therapy

C.A. Hackethal, M.D. has reported excellent success in treating Parkinson's Disease by use of replacement therapy of DHEA. Apparently the bad side-effects of L-Dopa are avoided, and the Parkinsonian victim is restored to appropriate functioning. As a collateral observation, Dr. Hackethal has observed Rheumatoid Disease patients (who also have Parkinson's Disease) become well even when C-reactive protein and Rh-factor is positive. This may be a linkage between loss of homeostatic hormones and the onset of Rheumatoid Disease, and conversely, this may also highlight the reason why replacement therapy of cortisone increases the rate of disease progress, as well as its other bad side effects on Rheumatoid Disease victims. But Parkinson's Disease and Rheumatoid Disease are only two of many health problems that DHEA may help in some way, including various geriatric and metabolic problems, Cancer, Diabetes, immune system enhancement, improved brain function, infection, obesity, Osteoporosis, Alzheimer's Disease, Chronic Fatigue Syndrome, and estrogen replacement[96,107].

According to Julian Whitaker, M.D.[96] "Blood levels of DHEA in men and women peak around age 20, and it is the only hormone that declines in a linear fashion in both sexes. As such it is one of the most reliable markers of aging. By age 80, blood levels of DHEA are only 5% of what they were at 20."

Dr. Julian Whitaker[107] says, "DHEA is extraordinarily safe. Administered by prescription, it is given in physiological replacement dosage (up to 90-100 mg per day, usually less, or up to 250 mg per day, according to some other physicians, depending upon age and need). You should find DHEA to be safer than most over-the-counter items such as Tylenol®, Sudafed®, Motrin®, or even aspirin, and far safer than almost all other prescription drugs.

"The goal of physiological replacement is to increase your blood level of DHEA or DHEA sulfate (both levels are comparable) to that found in a normal 20 to 30 year-old person. Therefore, if you are a 55 year-old who has a normal blood level of DHEA for your age, physiological replacement is used to increase your blood level to that of a younger, healthier individual. If your blood level of DHEA is equal to or lower than that of people in your age group, then your risk of disease and other consequences of aging is far higher than the health risks of physiological replacement therapy with DHEA.

"In general, your body tends to utilize the extra DHEA if it needs it, and ignores it if it doesn't. For instance, if DHEA is given to an animal with a viral infection, the animal will use all the extra DHEA to enhance its immune system. If the animal does not have a viral infection, the extra DHEA is simply ignored.

"Prescribing and using DHEA is both legal and rational. But because it is an unpatentable therapy, the FDA takes the stance that it is `experimental,' and has been overcontrolling it for years. ... Since no drug company can patent it, the FDA denies you access to it, giving drug companies a clear shot at making metabolites of DHEA that they can patent."

Hydrogen Peroxide Therapy and Ozone Therapy

Hydrogen Peroxide has been in medical use for several centuries[34,37,39], and there are thousands of scientific studies on its use. What is not well known is that Hydrogen Peroxide is also used by many both internally[37] and externally for many different disease conditions, including Rheumatoid Disease. Ozone Therapy[35] is somewhat newer on the medical scene. These two are often referred to as "Oxygen Therapies," which is somewhat of a misnomer. One can take a breath of air and receive more oxygen than one can receive from Hydrogen Peroxide Therapy, and the use of Ozone Therapy[32]. Although not entirely understood, these two therapies clearly do not supply significant additional oxygen. In applying Ozone Therapy, like Photopheresis, a certain supply of blood is removed, treated with Ozone, and then replaced in the patient.

In desperation for relief -- any kind of relief -- arthritics will gradually increase their oral intake of food-grade hydrogen peroxide, many reporting relief of their symptoms, and sometimes their degenerative conditions.

Other physicians, including Charles H. Farr, M.D., Ph.D.[31], have shown that the intravenous usage of hydrogen peroxide has a beneficial effect on many disease states. Dr. Farr has also shown that the good effects of intravenous hydrogen peroxide usage stem principally from its ability to activate oxidation enzymes.

Miscellaneous Treatments

Osteoarthritis and Rheumatoid Arthritis have been historically viewed by traditional medical practitioners as two far-ranging "unsolved" disease conditions. As established medicine admits to no answer despite a multitude of modern scientific tests and categorizations of phenomena, it is not surprising to find that trial and error medicine by those concerned and those afflicted have brought about some practical answers. What is surprising is that many of these answers have no clear or clearly known underlying basis. For example, among various proffered solutions to either the inflammatory conditions, or to the underlying unknown physiological mechanisms, are Diet, Extreme Cold Therapy, Hydrotherapy, Poultices and Topical Treatments, Homeopathy, modern methods based on Professor Dr. Guenther Enderlein's work[68], Biomagnetics, Colon Therapy, Sound Therapy, Color Therapy, Aromatherapy, Mental Healing, Ayurveda, Dental Involvement (replacing poisonous mercury amalgams), Live Cell Therapy, Hydrogen Peroxide Therapy, Acupuncture, Acupressure, Rolfing, Oxygen and Ozone Therapy, Photopheresis, Yoga, Chelation Therapy[98] and many specialized organic substances from either the land[61] or sea[36]. Obviously not all of these treatments work for 100% of the afflicted or there would be no reason for this book.

The Rheumatoid Disease Foundation takes the position that -- since traditional medicine admits to no answers -- each person must search out the medical answer for him/herself, and that search may require open-mindedly trying one recommendation after another. After all, to the afflicted, it is not the correct theory that is important, but whether or not desirable results are achieved.

Chapter IV
Rheumatoid Arthritis
What Causes Rheumatoid Arthritis?
There are several hypotheses as to the cause of Rheumatoid Arthritis, among which are (1) a defective immunological system, and (2) a genetic susceptibility to the antigens of a foreign protein, or toxin, usually ascribed to microorganisms, such as bacteria, protozoa, yeast/fungus, mycoplasma, and virus. Both of these hypotheses

are acceptable, but only the first receives the majority of funding from pharmaceutical companies who have an interest in convincing that their patented immuno-modulating drugs are better than someone else's. Other hypotheses include an unbalanced hormonal system[85] and/or nutritional factors[1]. Corazon Ilarina, M.D.[40] based her medical practice on an idea that toxins are "trapped" in collagen (connective) tissue, and that these toxins may be from virus, bacteria, fungus, chemicals, foods and drugs.

There is considerable scientific medical evidence that Cell Wall Deficient microorganisms are found in many different kinds of joint diseases. These include variants of Gonococci, Staphylococci, Clostridia, Salmonella, Listeria, Mycoplasma, Virus, Corynebacteria and Propionibacteria. And these variants are found in Recurrent Staphylococcal Osteomyelities, Chronic Staphylococcal Osteomyelitis, Streptococcal Osteomyelitis, Listeria Osteomyelitis, Sclerosing Osteomyelitis, Pyoarthrosis, Gonococcal Arthritis, Clostridial Arthritis, Salmonella Arthritis, Staphylococcal Arthritis, Septic Arthritis of Children, Hemophilus Influenzae Arthritis, Mycobacterial Arthritis, Nocardia Asteroides in Canine Arthritis, Streptococcal Arthritis, Juvenile Rheumatoid Arthritis, Spondylitis and so on[77].

If the truth were wholly known, we would probably find that Rheumatoid Arthritis is a manifestation of the body mal-adapting to multiple causes, among which are (1) a weakened immunological system, (2) a developed internal allergic response to unknown allergens, including food allergens, or toxins[38], (3) Candidiasis, (4) external allergies[38], (5) lack of appropriate nutrition, including vitamins and minerals, (6) hormonal factors, (7) stress, and (8) other unknown factors[2].

Until the discovery of the Syphilis spirochete

(*Treponema pallidum*), Syphilis would have been classified as an ideal example of a defective immunological system — just as many Rheumatologists now view Rheumatoid Disease[1,2]. Prior to the discovery of the Tubercle bacillus (*Mycobacterium tuberculosis*), there were perhaps 100 different names (and therefore presumed to be 100 different diseases) for external symptoms observed by physicians. After the discovery of the Syphilis spirochete and the Tubercle bacillus — single source-causations — Syphilis was no longer viewed as a defect of the immuological system and those one hundred Tuberculosis names collapsed into one name: Tuberculosis of the spine, of the lung, of the skin, of the bone, and so on[1, 2].

Historically, according to Professor Roger Wyburn-Mason, M.D., Ph.D., Rheumatoid Disease seems to model itself after both Syphilis and Tuberculosis in that nearly all pharmaceutical research is aimed at proving that the individual's immunological system is defective and therefore needs modulated by some drug that damages the immunological system even further; and also in that there have been created many different names on the physician's viewing of differing symptoms, but in fact all belonging to the same disease process. Seldom are the named diseases found pure and isolated, but rather there will be components of many named diseases found in the same patient, indicating that the underlying commonality is collagen tissue disease, now newly named under the cluster heading of Rheumatoid Disease[1,29].

Rheumatoid Diseases are collagen tissue diseases. Collagen tissue is pervasive throughout the body and the disease, therefore, affects every portion of the anatomy including, but not limited to, periarteritis, Paget's Disease, cysts, myelomas, tremors, seizures, bronchitis, intrinsic asthma, dysrhythmias, myocardial disease, pericardial disease, appendicitis, mesenteric adentitis, ulcerative colitis, thyroid, parathyroid, thymus, pituitary, adrenal, gonads, atropic mucosa (pernicious anemia), webs, iridocyclitis, exophthalmias, bursitis, ovarian cysts, fibroids, salpingitis-sterility, tubal pregnancies, neuroses, psychoses, senility, systemic lupus erythematosus[14], polycythemia, purpura, arthritis, pyelonephritis, calculi, hepatitis, cholangitis, gallbladder disease, regional enterities, Crohn's disease, alveolitis, lymphomas, splenomegaly, headache, meningomas, myositis, trigeminal neuralgia, multiple sclerosis, rhinitis, eustachian salpingitis, enlarged tonsils, and adenoids, fetal deformities, abortions, pancreatitis, maturity diabetes, noninsulin dependent diabetes, SICCA syndrome, psoriasis[15], alopecia, erythemas, urticaria, degenerated discs, low back syndrome, tendonitis, ganglion, and coealic disease[1,29].

Prevention Of Rheumatoid Arthritis

There are several primary keys known to effectively prevent Rheumatoid Arthritis with most people, although it is also true that embryos and newly born children (Still's disease) can be affected by unknown mechanisms or by means of circumstances beyond their control. Among these primary keys, of course, are the dual mechanisms of insuring proper diet[62,63] and vitamin[64], mineral and essential fatty acid supplements, and relief from stressful living conditions[1,2].

Gus J. Prosch, Jr., M.D. Diet

One biochemical specialist on nutrition stated that folks place two kinds of objects in their mouths. One is called "food", and the other is called "nonfood". He said he'd explain what "nonfood" is first. That "nonfood" is anything that has been packaged, processed, refined, canned, dried, frozen, or has been changed from its original condition in any way. "`Food," he said, "is what you get out of the garden."

Like many other holistically oriented physicians, Gus J. Prosch, Jr., M.D.[95], recommends use of unpolluted fresh vegetables and fruits, whole grains and nuts, cold water fish (for essential fatty acids), and so on.

Dr. Prosch[2] says, "I would like to discuss the importance of diet, nutrition and vitamin and mineral supplementation in Rheumatoid Disease patients. Many different opinions and conclusions among most physicians today are fairly rampant and many doctors do not believe this subject is important, so I'm going to tell you about my beliefs and observations as to how and why I treat my patients, but I want to stress that these methods are my own opinions.

"In my observations and research there are several things that to me stand out to be quite significant in most patients with Rheumatoid Disease.

"1. The great majority of Rheumatoid Disease patient's body fluids are too acid in nature.

"2. The great majority of these patients show signs and symptoms of a deficiency in free or ionic calcium.

"3. Most Rheumatoid Disease patients eat margarine instead of butter and they demonstrate a lack of Vitamin A and natural D-3 plus severe deficiencies of the essential fatty acids.

"4. Diet in Rheumatoid Disease does help control the severity of the symptoms.

"5. Vitamin and mineral supplementations help shorten the recovery time by strengthening the immune system.

"In studying the nutrition status and diet of Rheumatoid Disease patients, I made three observations that have caused me to look deeper into this subject.

"1. I observed that many patients who are blood-related to arthritic patients do not develop any arthritis especially when different dietary habits were followed.

"2. I observed that often-times arthritic patients exhibited slight to significant improvement when self-administered home and folk remedies were taken, like alfalfa tablets, bone meal tablets, cod liver oil, vinegar with honey, peanut oil, . . . or cherries.

"3. I observed that some arthritic patients are more susceptible to getting reinfected after being treated with the medication that apparently eliminated the offending organisms. I found by checking the acidity of saliva and urine of arthritic patients, that the great majority were considerably more acid than normal and I concluded that an alkaline diet could only benefit these patients.

"I also found by careful observation that Rheumatoid Disease patients more often than normal exhibited certain physical signs during the physical examination. To summarize these signs, they are as follows:

"1. Longitudinal ridges and increased opaqueness in fingernails.

"2. Mild to moderate tenderness with strong palpation of the soleus or trapezius muscles.

"3. Generalized slight increase in deep tendon reflexes.

"4. Generalized irritability of skeletal muscles to percussion.

"5. Acid saliva of pH 4.5 to 6.5.

"6. Slight to severe coating on the tongue.

"Many of these signs are related to calcium metabolism in the body and most arthritic patients drink 2% or low fat milk and eat margarine instead of butter.

"The previously mentioned physical signs demonstrate strong evidence of free or ionic calcium deficiency as well as a deficiency of Vitamin A and D_3 which is natural Vitamin D. Blood calcium studies are misleading as they measure the ionic calcium as well as calcium bound to proteins. Whereas normal body fluids ideally are slightly alkaline as opposed to acid, and I believe the one primary cause of the deficiency in Rheumatoid Disease patients is the ionic calcium which in itself is very alkaline.

"An even more important cause of this acidity is due to the diet and nutritional habits of these arthritic patients. Most cellular mechanisms of the body and particularly those involving the use of ionized minerals such as the secretory glands, nerve function processes and muscle contraction, etc. proceed best in a mildly alkaline state. For this reason a diet consisting of high alkaline foods should be consumed, combined with the avoidance of acid forming foods. Acid forming foods are those which are high in one or more of three elements: phosphorus, sulfur and chlorine; alkaline forming foods are those which are high in one or more the four elements, potassium, calcium, magnesium and sodium. The diet used to treat and prevent development of Rheumatoid Diseases should definitely avoid as much as possible the following foods. All processed and most canned foods should be avoided along with caffeine, sugar in all it's forms, as well as the simple carbohydrate foods that quickly upon digestion turn into sugar, like white flour foods, crackers, many cereals, macaroni (pasta foods) white rice and corn products. Ideally nicotine and alcohol should be avoided, along with any sweets, candy, soft drinks, pastries and desserts. The `nightshade plants' (foods containing solanines) such as white potatoes, tomatoes, egg plant and garden peppers should be avoided. (Robert Bingham, M.D. states that about 1/3 of arthritics are affected by solanines: Ed.).

"As a rule, most protein foods tend to be acid forming since they contain phosphorus and sulfur. Animal sources of protein — lean meat (beef, lamb, veal) poultry, fish and eggs — are definitely in this category. With the exception of shrimp, most sea food is extremely acid forming. These foods must not be avoided however in the diet, as they provide the building blocks for all body functions and processes. Therefore one of these proteins should be eaten with each meal. Pork meats should be limited however. Just try not to eat an entire meal consisting of protein foods, but balance these foods with alkaline forming foods. Ideally your breakfast should always consist of some high protein foods, balanced with whole milk, fruit juices, etc. Also remember to cook protein foods at low temperatures, as enzymes and trace minerals are reduced with excessive heat and no foods should be eaten that have been deep fried.

"Avoid processed and hydrogenated, or `hardened' oils and fats. Most margarines, peanut butters, restaurant prepared french fries and potato or corn chips are prepared with hardened oils. Sweet cream butter is best and use `cold pressed' vegetable oils or `Pam' for home cooking. Also watch those high calorie salad dressings. Most fats and fatty foods (butter, oils, sausages, bacon, etc.) are neutral in their acid-alkaline content but they greatly contribute to excessive weight gain which severely complicates arthritis. Therefore, it would be wise to limit all oily, greasy, fried, fatty foods if one tends to be overweight.

"Most all vegetables (except corn) are highly alkaline in nature and should be emphasized in the eating program. Salad vegetables are excellent and should be eaten daily. All other vegetables are very good and when `Wok' cooked or stir fried in cold pressed vegetable oil are even better.

"Fresh vegetable juices (not canned) are nearly perfect and should be part of the diet. It is important to prepare and serve as many foods in their raw and natural state as possible.

"All fruits and fruit juices (excepting cranberries, plums and prunes) are alkaline forming and are good to `munch' on.

"Whole milk is one of the best alkaline forming foods due to its high calcium content. Raw certified whole milk is much preferable if you can find it. At least two glasses of whole milk should be taken each day and use butter instead of margarine. Plain yogurt is an excellent alkalinizing food and not only is easy to digest, but tastes great when mixed with fresh fruit such as raisins, dates, dried figs and apricots. It also makes excellent munching foods.

"This diet will change one's system to be more alkaline as it should be.

"Concerning vitamin and mineral supplementation, the most important point to consider here is to correct the free calcium deficiency present in most arthritics. This requires much larger amounts of vitamin A and D in their natural form than what is usually recommended by the `Recommended Daily Allowances' tables.

"The synthetic Vitamin A and D-2 preparations on the market simply do not work. Synthetic Vitamin D-2 does increase the calcium absorption from the small intestine but seems to be totally inadequate in regulating the use of the calcium and especially calcium excretion by the kidneys. The only preparation I have found that is adequate is the natural D-3 which is found in fish liver oils. Therefore I recommend Norwegian Cod Liver Oil as the ideal which seems to be even better than cod liver oil capsules. It is easily taken when mixed with some orange juice and stirred rapidly. The preparation I recommend is plain Norwegian Cod Liver Oil liquid which contains 10,000 units of Vitamin A and 1000 units of Vitamin D per teaspoon. I recommend that patients take two teaspoons on arising each morning and two teaspoons at bedtime. This preparation can be found in most health food stores and should be taken for at least four months, then the dosage should be cut in half.

"I explain to the patients not to fear any Vitamin A or D toxicity with this dosage as it is less than 1/3 the toxicity level that has been reported in the literature. If the patient absolutely cannot take the liquid, they can usually find capsules at a health food store which will provide approximately 4,000 units of Vitamin D daily.

"I also explain that exposure to sunshine for at least 20 minutes each week will activate the Vitamin D.

"Concerning the calcium preparations I have found that none of the available inorganic calcium preparations are effective. I discovered that organic bone meal tablets (3-4 per day) work better than other calcium preparations but I continued to have reservations. Recently I located a calcium preparation which seems to work ideally. It is the naturally occurring calcium in plants. I prescribe 500 mg. This compound is Calcium Orotate (500 mg 4 times daily).

"This calcium preparation also seems to enhance the ability of the body to use and metabolize other forms of calcium ingested.

"I also prescribe 500 mg of Magnesium Orotate [or Magnesium Aspartate: Ed.] twice daily to balance the calcium/magnesium ratio. The above calcium preparation is also excellent for osteoporosis and it greatly strengthens the bone and cartilage structures in the body. [While not the ideal, Ca/Mg aspartate may be substituted if the orotate is not available: Ed.]

"Concerning other vitamins for arthritic patients, I recommend as an ideal supplemental program the following:

"a. Vitamin B Complex, two to three `Stress' B vitamins daily in divided doses. (These should contain 50-

75 mg of each B vitamin).

"b. Vitamin C, two to three grams daily in divided doses.

"c. Zinc Orotate, 500 mg one to two tablets on an empty stomach. [Zinc Gluconate; Zinc Picolinate or some other acceptable form: Ed.]

"d. Selenium, 250 micrograms daily as yeast selenium.

"e. B-Carotene, 25,000 units daily.

"f. Vitamin E, 400 units daily.

"The above vitamin and mineral supplementations will not only help the patient's arthritis by stimulating the immune response system but will play an important role in counteracting the aging process as well as acting as a deterrent to some forms of cancer since many of these preparations act as free radical and peroxide scavengers in the body.

"With painful hands and feet, I recommend in addition 100 mg Vitamin B-6."

Carl J. Reich, M.D. Diet

Dr. Prosch's experienced recommendations regarding acidity/alkalinity and calcium deficiency for arthritis, were initially discovered by Carl J. Reich, M.D.[102] of Canada, in 1950, who, over many years of clinical practice and research, concluded that the object, for wellness, is to insure that bodily tissues are sustained as an alkaline, as opposed to an acidic condition, and this can be tested easily by a simple litmus paper test on saliva that is free from food and drinks momentarily. A litmus paper test of small children, then older children, and so on upwards toward older adults, will demonstrate that litmused saliva tends to be very dark purplish and then slowly fade out as an acid condition takes over from inappropriate nourishment as we age[1,2]. Our pH saliva test should be slightly alkaline, or dark blue. Seldom is this true of the arthritic.

"By 1958, after observing and treating thousands of patients, Dr. Reich definitely concluded that chronic disease such as asthma, ileitis and colitis were not the results of the direct effect of ionic calcium deficiency on the lung and intestinal tract. Instead he concluded that these diseases were the indirect result of deficiency and represented the breakdown of autonomically excited adaptive function in an attempt to compensate for its deficient state. Thus, Dr. Reich believed that deficiency of certain nutrients caused the organs to become more vulnerable to disease. He began to look on cases of angina (heart pain to the chest caused by overexertion of a diseased heart) as "asthma of the systemic arteries;" and on forms of ileitis and colitis (inflammation of the lower intestine and colon respectively) as "asthma of the intestinal tract," and to treat them with preparations containing calcium and vitamin-D, exactly as he had treated his first cases of bronchial asthma[102]."

Over a period of many years Dr. Reich concluded that most chronic disease, such as cancer and arthritides, was a maladaptation to lack of sufficient ionic calcium at the cellular level. His recommendation, which helped many to restore their health, was the use of calcium and other vitamins and mineral supplements in excess of RDA allowances, but also particularly large quantities of Vitamin D and sunshine to activate the Vitamin D, which then permits the calcium to be utilized[102]. Dr. Reich's recommendations follow[102]:

Schedule of Initial Daily Dosages of Vitamins and Minerals[102]

Patient	-----------Daily Dosage -------------		
(Age)	Vitamin-A (I.U.)	Vitamin-D (I.U.)	Calcium
	(milligrams)		
3-6	5,000 to 8,000	1,000 to 2,400	250 to 500
15	30,000	4,800	750
Adult	54,000	7,200	1,250

"These are maintained for several weeks or months and then reduced to one-half to one-third[102].

1. Dosage given was an average number that adjusted slightly up or down depending on weight.

2. About half the dosages of vitamin-A and vitamin-D was given in the form of halibut liver oil, and half in water soluble form, "Aquasol A and D[102]."

Some Patients Treated with Vitamins and Minerals by Dr. Carl Reich[102]

Type of Disease (Acidic Saliva pH)	Number of Patients	Good to Excellent Resolution
Adult Chronic Asthma	5,000	67%
Child Chronic Asthma	6,000	93%
Rheumatoid Arthritis	100	60%
Osteoarthritis	2,000	60%

Dr. Reich says, "The basis of the importance of ionic Ca^{++} in health is that we evolved under a blanket of solar radiation which simultaneously photosynthesized the following four compounds in vegetable and living cells, and no others. These were glucose, oxygen, vitamin D and melanin. Therefore calcium which that vitamin ionized was destined to be intimately related to the energizing of the cell, and its deficiency to give rise to cell energy starvation and adaptation to that deficiency starvation[102].

"The undertow common to the dragging down of most patients with major diseases is that which is due to adaptive functions of organs and tissue which have been autonomically excited on various organs such as lungs, intestines, arterial tree, skeleton, and the metabolizing tissue, to exert biochemical adaption to ionic calcium deficiency. The pressure of persisting life-style defects creating the deficiency, results in maladaptive disease such as asthma, ileitis-colitis, hypertension, arthritis, and diabetes. Secondary factors, such as the type of infection the patient contracts, other deficiencies, toxic excesses, genetic factors and others, dictate which organ or tissue will be called upon to perform this function. For reasons which the demand that they make on the same adaptive mechanisms, psychic or physical stress will hasten the onset of such disease and be mistakenly looked upon as the prime causative factor. The variety or combination of ionic calcium deficiency maladaptive disease which may afflict a person represents the variety of those secondary causes. Likewise the variety or combination of such diseases that may afflict the skeleton represents the variety of a subgroup of those causes[102]."

Niacinamide and Boron

As with the treatment of Osteoarthritis, joint conditions can be greatly improved through the usage of William Kaufman's (M.D., Ph.D.) regimen of niacinamide, the dosage dependent upon the degree of joint inflexibility as measured by a special easy-to-use scale[89, 90, 91]. Rex Newnham, Ph.D., D.O., N.D. and his Boron deficiency discoveries has also been reported under the section on Osteoarthritis[23]·

Vitamin C Therapy[2]

As the effects of Vitamin C are so very important for sustaining, and achieving health, Dr. Robert F. Cathcart,'s (M.D.) research findings and clinical use of Vitamin C should be repeatedly stressed. Vitamin C is the greatest single assist in fighting disease, strengthening the immune system, restoring after stress, supporting the activity of other vitamins and minerals, and many other good benefits[2]. Cathcart says: "Well nourished humans contain not much more than 5 grams of Vitamin C in their bodies. The majority of people have much less, and therefore are at risk for many problems related to failure of metabolic processes that depend on ascorbate. Irwin Stone calls this condition 'chronic subclinical scurvy'[2].

Linus Pauling, Ph.D., against great odds, has convinced rational physicians and scientists of the great importance of Vitamin C. His recent studies and conclusions lead him to believe that atherosclerosis is simply a symptom on the way to full-blown scurvy[98]. Irwin Stone, Fred R. Kenner, M.D. and many others have conducted so many thousands of studies demonstrating the importance of Vitamin C that there only remains the need to describe how it is to be used. Cathcart has done this in what is known as the Cathcart Bowel Tolerance Method[2].

As most mammals, including humans, do not have the ability to synthesize Vitamin C, it is imperative that our nutritional intake include substantial quantities of it. Routinely some folks, including the author, take 6 to 8 grams (in powered form) per day, not counting what is routinely obtained in vegetables and fruits[2].

Vitamin C can be taken either as an injectable (IV), if severely ill, or in oral form as Sodium Ascorbate, Calcium Ascorbate or Ascorbic acid. Generally its easier to take it in powered or crystalline form, dissolved in a fluid, than in the form of tablets. The reason is that the Cathcart Bowel Tolerance Method cannot be used when the Vitamin C is in tablet form, as the binders that hold the powder together will interfere with the phenomena that is to be observed[2].

According to Cathcart, a normal person can probably get by on between 4 and 15 grams per 24 hour period. When one comes down with a sickness, or has been under unusual stress, one increases the amount of Vitamin C consumed within 24 hours to the point where diarrhea just begins -- then one backs off to the dosage used just prior to the diarrhea. That "just lower than" figure is the exact amount your body needs for the time being[2].

It may be necessary to increase your dosages by amounts of 5, 10, 15, or greater grams per 24 hour period until you find the correct dosage. It's important to understand that different ill-health conditions require differing amounts of grams of Vitamin C per 24 hour period, and that this can vary from 4 grams on up to hundreds of grams that must be given via intravenous drip[2].

It is now routine to speak of a "50 gram cold", or "150 gram influenza", or a "50 gram allergy"[2]! The more infection, the more Vitamin C is required by the body.

Cathcart's use of Vitamin C covers colds, influenza, Coxsackievirus, mononucleosis, viral pneumonia, hay fever, asthma, food allergy, stress, cancer, ankylosing spondylitis, Reiter's syndrome, rheumatoid arthritis, bacterial infections, infectious hepatitis, Candidiasis, and other ailments[2].

Although the bowel tolerance method cannot be used for a new kind of Vitamin C, ESTER-C™, may be a preferred form because of its ability to enter the blood stream more rapidly, staying in the body longer, and circulating in larger quantities to all tissues. ESTER-C is manufactured by Inter-Cal Corporation in Prescott, Arizona, and was first reported in the professional literature by Anthony J. Verlangieri, Ph.D. of the Atherosclerosis Research Laboratories at the University at Mississippi. He demonstrated that ESTER-C "entered the bloodstream in half the time, doubled the amount of vitamin C entering the blood and doubled the time that the nutrient was circulating through the body." Verlangieri also compared ESTER-C against calcium ascorbate, finding that calcium ascorbate was absorbed at only "one-half the level of ESTER-C Calcium Polyascorbate[103]."

Jonathan V. Wright, M.D. conducted a human utilization study demonstrating that ESTER-C "wasted only one-third as much as ordinary vitamin C and sent four times more to the tissue level[103]."

ESTER-C Calcium Polyascorbate is well worth investigating for daily usage.

Magnesium Chloride Therapy[85]

Raul Vergini,M.D.[85] reported on the past medical history of the good effects of the use of Magnesium Chloride for many different conditions, including, but not limited to: colitis, angiocholitis, cholecystitis, in the digestive system, senile tremor, Parkinson's disease, muscular cramps, for the nervous system, acne, eczema, psoriasis, warts, itch, chilblains, strengthening of hair and nails, diseases of the aged (impotency, prostatic hypertrophy, cerebral and circulatory troubles), allergies (hayfever, asthma, urticaria, anaphylactic reactions, cancer, and so on.)

Dr. Vergini has within recent years verified many of these uses for magnesium chloride hexahydrate used orally or intravenously. His personal experience includes good effects in the treatment of herpes zoster, acute and chronic conjunctivitis, optic neuritis, rheumatic diseases, many allergic diseases, spring-asthenia, and Chronic Fatigue Syndrome.

He says that, "the solution to be used is a 2.5%

Magnesium Chloride hexahydrate ($MgCl_2.6H_2O$) solution (25 grams/1 liter of water).

"Dosages are as follows:

Adults and children over 5	125cc
4 year old children	100cc
3 year old children	80cc
1-2 year old children	30cc
Under 6 month old children	15cc

"These doses must be administered *by mouth*. For chronic diseases the standard treatment is one dose morning and evening for a long period.

"In acute diseases the dose is administered every 6 hours (every 3 hours the first two doses if the case is serious); then spaced every 8 hours and then 12 hours as improvement goes on. After recovery it's better to continue with a dose every 12 hours for some days. As a preventive measure, and as a magnesium supplement, one dose a day can be taken. Magnesium chloride, even if it's an inorganic salt, is very well absorbed and it's a very good supplemental magnesium source.

"For *intravenous* injection the formula is:

Magnesium chloride hexahydrate 25 grams

Distilled water 100cc

"Make injections of 10-20cc (over 10-20 minutes) once or twice a day. Of course the solution must be sterilized[85]."

Chelation Therapy[98]

*(References in this chapter are found
at the end of the section.)*

What is Chelation Therapy?

Pronounced "Key-lay'-shun," Chelation Therapy is one of the most effective treatments for a wide spectrum of diseases or aging conditions. But it is more than a treatment, it is a preventive process and most certainly a treatment of the 21st century effectively practiced by many physicians today. It is the only therapy where physicians who practice it habitually use it on themselves and their loved ones as either curative or preventive treatment. Critics of Chelation Therapy have never used it on themselves, nor their loved ones, nor on their patients, nor have they read the voluminous literature that has been compiled by various physicians and scientists who are members of the American College of Advancement in Medicine[1] (ACAM), an organization dedicated to certification in the practice of Chelation Therapy and to further its research.

In Chelation Therapy, the imagery is often used of the lobster claw, grabbing onto a cation -- a positive metal ion -- in the blood stream during the process of surrounding a positive (metal) ion. The chemical equivalent of the lobster claw is a protein, an amino acid called EDTA (Ethylene Diamine Tetracetic Acid). EDTA combines with cations in the blood stream, flushing them out with urine. Do not think, however, that this is the only form of chelation that can take place within the body. The most common form of chelation is that which takes place during strenuous exercise, producing lactic acid, a natural chelator.

According to James J. Julian, M.D.[2] "Chelation is a basic process of life itself. Without the chelation mechanism, life as we know it would not exist on this planet.

"Chelation is the process that enables plants to take inorganic elements and change them into organic plant structure. Chlorophyll of green plants is a chelate of the mineral magnesium; blood hemoglobin (the oxygen carrier) is a chelate of iron. Chelation is the process by which the body utilizes aspirin, penicillin, vitamins, minerals and trace elements."

Chelation is a natural process found in nature. Soap is

a chelator, taking off grime and dirt. When you soften water through a house water-softener, you use a chelating agent to take out minerals. EDTA, when used in your 100,000 miles of internal plumbing called capillaries, veins and arteries, acts in a similar manner, by taking out metal ions that will otherwise damage us[7].

As Julian[2] further explains, "A modified copy of one of these natural amino acids called ethylene diamine tetracetic acid (EDTA), is used in Chelation Therapy. It is modified to make it more predictable and dependable in removing specific elements with [positive] electric charges such as calcium and heavy metals; namely lead, arsenic, mercury, cadmium and aluminum from the body."

In 1893, Swiss Nobel Laureate Alfred Werner proposed a theory of metal which provided the foundation for modern chelation therapy[10,11]. In the early 1930's Germany and the United States both experimented with chemical processes for synthesizing EDTA[11]. Chelation therapy was first used by the British in WWII as an antidote to poison gas inhalation. According to John Parks Trowbridge, M.D. and Morton Walker, "The earliest reported research using EDTA for removal of plaque-producing calcium deposits was conducted in 1946 at the University of Zurich, and in 1947 and 1948 at the University of Bern[39]." In 1948 the U.S. Navy used EDTA to treat lead poisoning. Dr. Norman E. Clarke, Director of Research at Providence Hospital in Detroit, observed that after a series of treatments with EDTA, patients' overall health appeared to improve. Patients who had angina reported that their chest pain was gone. Others with gangrene of the legs reported healing. Memory, sight, hearing and sense of smell all improved. People treated with chelation reported increased vigor[11].

Clarke's observations stirred up interest in physicians who reported a wide-range of benefits to patients suffering from heart disease, brain disorders, and arteriosclerosis. It was clear that EDTA was effective not only in removing toxic metals, but also in helping restore blood vessels blocked by placque.

In 1952 W. Grant, M.D., in a research paper, "described the use of EDTA chelation therapy as a solution for removing calcium from the eyes of human patients with post-keratitis corneal opacities which had resulted in cataracts[39]."

During the 1960's there was demonstrated a wide-range of benefits to patients suffering from various diseases. These demonstrations included both human and animal studies. In particular, "That EDTA is able to remove calcium from the arterial wall was conclusively shown in a study by Fred Walker, Ph.D. and outlined in his doctoral thesis[39]." But, a serious blow to EDTA study occurred in 1969 when a patient expired. This resulted in reduced motivation to establish the positive effects of EDTA in cardiovascular and age-associated diseases[11].

During the 1970's there were numerous medical/legal battles surrounding chelation therapy. Some MD's were placed on probation by their State Medical Boards. (This battle continues in certain states to this day.) Others have won battles which allowed them to use EDTA, which was approved by the FDA for metal toxicity. Other State Medical Boards either ignored the dispute, or tacitly approved the use of Chelation Therapy. Chelation Therapy is a treatment not generally accepted by the general medical establishment. In those few states where medical boards have closed down or prosecuted physicians who practice Chelation Therapy, the State Medical Boards for the most part consist of well-meaning physicians who are concerned with our welfare (and their own pocketbooks in some cases), but who know absolutely nothing about the therapy other than what they've read that was written by others who knew nothing about it. It is safe to say that every article written against Chelation Therapy and printed in "respectable" journals has been written by a physician or researcher who has assumed the mantle of Authority, yet has absolutely no knowledge of it. A presumed exception is a study performed by Danish surgeons (with conflict of interest) and published in the 1991 *American Journal of Surgery* and in the *Journal of Internal Medicine* 231:261-267 1992. It is clear from an analysis performed by the American Institute of Medical Preventics[44] that this study was either done in total ignorance of the appropriate methodology of scientific studies or, most probably, was fraudulently designed to cast aspersions against this otherwise wholly successful treatment for financial gain. Contrary to widespread opinion, neither science nor the field of medical practice is free of fraud, dishonesty and incompetence.

In 1973 the American Academy of Medical Preventics (now the American College of Advancement in Medicine [ACAM]) developed a safe and effective protocol for this therapy. Since that time more than half a million people have been helped according to documented case histories, "most of them victims of hardening of the arteries[39]." According to James P. Frackelton, President of the American Institute of Medical Preventics (AIMP), AIMP "is the holder of an Investigational New Drug permit issued by the U.S. Food and Drug Administration and is cosponsor of [an] ongoing FDA approved stud[y] of EDTA chelation therapy to treat atherosclerotic peripheral vascular disease with claudication. AIMP works closely with FDA officials to ensure that the studies are meticulously conducted, and that all FDA requirements can be met. If and when the studies are successful, the FDA would then approve atherosclerosis to be listed on the package insert of MgEDTA[45]."

This therapy historically began with the use of Calcium EDTA as a treatment for lead poisoning, called plumbism, after the chemical name for lead, plumbum. If you remember history, you'll recall that the Roman Empire was gifted with great engineers, and those engineers created a gigantic system of water plumbing made of lead. Some historians have hypothesized that lead poisoning from water contacting tubes of lead, and dissolving lead compounds, was a contributing factor to the downfall of the Roman Empire.

But you don't have to go as far back as the Roman Empire to observe lead poisoning. It was only rather recently that the U.S. Government banned lead from automotive gasoline engines, and also from interior paints which have poisoned so many children who have unwittingly eaten peeling lead paint.

Various doctors have been called upon from time to time to use Calcium EDTA chelation to rid a patient of lead poisoning acquired by one means or another, such as inhaling the fumes from the burning of lead batteries. In this process, the physician inserts a needle into the bloodstream and "pushes" a one-shot substance into the veins in the recognition that a chelating chemical will grab onto poisonous lead in the body, surround it, and allow the body to flush the poison out with the patient's urine.

That's the extent of knowledge that most physicians have about Chelation Therapy. If you ask them if they know anything about Chelation Therapy, they'll say "Yes!" thinking that you mean this single-push process developed in 1948 for ridding the body of excessive lead. Some fewer physicians will know of the use of flushing out bone-attractive materials such as plutonium.

EDTA Chelation Therapy described herein is gentler than the one-shot lead "push" and in many ways more beneficial. EDTA can surround, combine with and flush out many unwanted substances, such as calcium, lead, arsenic, aluminum and, indeed, any positive ion that is undesired and capable of being combined with this amino acid. Calcium EDTA is usually used for lead poisoning, whereas disodium EDTA is usually used in the described Chelation Therapy. Magnesium EDTA is being used with increasing frequency. At the termination of infusion of disodium EDTA, Calcium Gluconate is often placed in the infusion bottle, converting the remainder of the EDTA to Calcium EDTA, to help prevent calcium tetany. However Calcium, disodium and Magnesium EDTA are all suitable for their various purposes. Gordon E. Potter, M.D. reports that while EDTA is excellent for bivalent ions, Desferroxamine is superior for chelating out trivalent ions such as Iron (Fe^{+++}) and Aluminum (Al^{+++}). Since Desferroxamine passes through the blood brain barrier, it may also be superior for Alzheimer's disease; i.e. in chelating out aluminum[46]. EDTA and Desferroxamine may be used simultaneously, according to some physicians. According to Warren M. Levin, M.D." EDTA binds mercury avidly *in vitro* (in the test tube), but is ineffective *in vivo* (in the human body)[47]."

There are many poisons that we breathe in, eat, drink or are exposed to by bodily contact and skin absorption. The subject of environmental pollution is entirely too big to describe here, but everyone who reads newspapers, watches television, or hears radio will surely know that our bodies are currently bathed in undesirable pollutants of every kind. EDTA Chelation Therapy cannot rid us of everything foreign, of course, but it does an excellent job of chelating out many undesirable pollutants.

How Does Chelation Therapy Work?
While EDTA Chelation Therapy will "flush out" many undesirable substances, a chief effect is to contact, com-

bine with and to flush out calcium that is found in plaques in the arteries.

The molecules and atoms that "seek" out or have a very strong affinity for, other compounds and atoms are called "free radicals." Free radicals are always formed within the body as a natural consequence of a balance between catabolism and anabolism, the building up and breaking down of cellular tissue, respectively. Free radicals also have a vital place in killing foreign microorganism. Whenever the balance is seriously upset, and especially for extended periods, when more free radicals are formed than can be balanced off by natural bodily processes, disease and often accompanying inflammation occurs. Chelation Therapy has a definite place in the ridding of free-radicals that cause inflammation. It performs other duties that permit functioning for health, such as ridding the body of toxic pollutants which interfere with enzymal functions. Chelation Therapy operates at a level that is basic for the health of individual cells -- optimally functioning cells promote optimally functioning organs, and these, in turn, optimally functioning systems -- and consequent health. Because virtually all diseases have some component of production of an excess of free-radicals, Chelation Therapy can be and often is indicated as curative or supportive for many disease states, especially chronic diseases. Oxygen atoms and other chemicals within the body are attracted to other compounds and atoms forming free radicals during combinatorial stages. Free radicals damage tissues and promote cartilage decomposition and many other cascading problems for organs, systems and tissues generally. In addition, cells cannot eliminate their waste products. Cellular breakdown occurs leading to deterioration and disease. Over time, the entire arterial system is slowly disturbed, as are organs and tissues, all of them composed of individual cells with lowered reserves and capacities.

There are two explanations for the way EDTA Chelation Therapy works. Probably both theories or explanations are correct. One theory is the free radical theory; the other is the calcium binding theory, the removal of calcium that binds together the ingredients of plaques in our arteries.

Free Radical Theory

According to the free radical theory, perhaps 80-90% of all disease process is an excess of free radical activity[11,12,13,14,15]. Excessive free radicals create havoc by damaging cells and their DNA, changing biochemicals, damaging cell membranes and sometimes killing cells outright. Every oxygen factor also has an antioxidant factor in our physiological systems. We, in other words, are normally capable of neutralizing the harmful effects of atoms and molecules that have a high affinity for other elements and chemicals, and would otherwise damage tissue and cells in attaching to cellular components.

Whenever one side or the other of this oxidation/antioxidation, free-radical system becomes unbalanced, damage accrues. This damage leads to diseases of the circulatory system, malignancies, inflammatory conditions and immunologic disorders[13]. According to Elmer Cranton, M.D., "The free radical concept explains contradictory epidemiologic and clinical observations and provides a scientific rationale for treatment and prevention of many of the major causes of long-term disability and death: atherosclerosis, dementia, cancer, arthritis, and other age-related diseases[22]."

EDTA chelation therapy removes metals that act as catalysts for the production of excessive free radical reactions, thus halting the disease process and/or repairing the damage. Cranton says that "EDTA can reduce the production of free radicals by a million-fold[24]."

Calcium Binding Theory

A proper diet can also act as a chelator. "The proper program of low-fat, high-complex-carbohydrate diet and aerobic exercise actually is partially a natural process of chelation therapy.[23]" Specific foods and combinations of foods can, then, act as partial chelators. The extent and distribution of these foods would be too lengthy for this volume. However, as an example, specific studies have been completed on the chelating effects of garlic which show that garlic has a chelating effect on those suffering excessive lipid deposits. Benjamin Lau, M.D., Ph.D., who has accomplished a great deal of research on garlic, shows that the ratio of Low Density Lipids to Very Low Density Lipids decreased in a study over a period of six months using a particular form of aged garlic, 1 gram per day. At the same time, with the same ingredients and same dosage, Cholesterol also decreased. In both instances during an initial 60 day period, the measurable levels of lipids increased, which was interpreted as an initial sloughing off of the excessive lipid deposits, after which a continuous decrease was discovered[20].

Gradually, free radicals affect tissues so that localized accumulations of lipid-containing (oil/fat) material (atheromas) within or beneath the intima (lining of vessels) surfaces of blood vessels clog up the 100,000 miles of capillaries, veins and arteries[7]. Exposure to pollutants over a lifetime from food, air, water and drugs collect in various tissues throughout the body, in various ways. When EDTA chelates out many of these pollutants we find that we can now handle life better than before and we are healthier.

When EDTA binds with calcium, the consequence is the breakup of the plaque hindering the flow of blood in the arterial system. Probably, for many people, plaque formation in the arterial system begins sometime after birth about ages 4, 5 and 6 and continues onward until more than 50% of the system is plugged, and blood has a difficult time flowing, and thence disease conditions become evident. Military records show on autopsies from Korean and Vietnam conflicts that many United States' soldiers aged 18-25 had coronary artery disease[16]. Even two of the three pioneer astronauts who died in the notorious oxygen fire prior to takeoff -- three men picked for their excellent physical condition -- showed signs of atherosclerosis on autopsy.

There is a margin of safety built into every organ, and the circulatory system can compensate for increased demands for many years, until its flexibility and capacity is decreased to a critical limit.

In the calcium binding theory, calcium acts like a cement-binder, in that it binds fatty substances together, probably over a scar tissue, and forms the placque linings that cause the arterial system to decrease in flow volume. By Chelating out the calcium binder, the plaque dissolves and increases the diameter of the artery while also increasing the artery's flexibility.

When a fluid flows through a pipe or tube, the rate of flow depends on a number of factors, including the pipe's length, its radius, the fluid's viscosity and the time of flow. All other factors staying constant, a very small decrease or increase in the radius of the tube decreases or increases the rate of flow, respectively, by a factor of the power of three. Since a smaller vascular opening also requires higher blood pressure to pump the blood through, more work is placed on the heart and overall vascular system. With increased clogging of the circulatory system, therefore, our blood pressure increases while the quantity or volume of blood flow decreases drastically[8]. Since the human vascular system is not rigid, like metal pipes, the subject of cross-sectional diameter and fluid flow can be oversimplified, as the arteries may also stretch with higher pressure, therefore compensating to some extent for a smaller diameter of flow openings. However "perfusion scans have demonstrated increased brain blood flow after Chelation treatment . . . doppler ultrasound studies in sample groups of up to 30 patients have demonstrated some cases of complete patency [the condition of being wide open] of carotid arteries following treatment . . . [and] there is a 28% improvement or enlargement of the lumen [inner lining] diameter . . . improvement in brachial-ankle blood pressure ratios . . .[23]" and according to Zigurts Strauts, M.D. A 10% increase in vascular diameter of the arteries is enough to double the blood flow[43]."

As atherosclerosis progresses, and the pipes — the capillaries, arteries and veins — decrease in size, each cell of our body also receives considerably less nourishment than before partial clogging, as the amount of nourishment lessens with the decrease of blood flow. There is literally less opportunity to bring molecular food particles and oxygen to each cell. With less food and oxygen at each cell, the cell has less capacity to function. Less functioning of each cell means less ability to resist disease and stress, and less ability to repair damage already done. That, of course, means increased opportunity for every kind of disease[7]!

Ionic Calcium Deficiency Theory

A new explanation for the effectiveness of Chelation Therapy is based on the explanation of Carl J. Reich, M.D. and E.W. McDonagh, D.O., who report that "fringe benefits of chelation therapy likely represents the relief of the ionic calcium deficiency symptoms and diseases. This relief likely occurs because, as EDTA chelates molecular calcium out of metastatic deposits in arteries it naturally has to ionize it. In the process some goes to resolve the total body ionic calcium deficiency[102,105]."

How Are Treatments Given?

The chemical EDTA, an amino acid, acts like a magnet for positively charged calcium and other metal ions. The chemical EDTA "claws" onto the metallic ions and converts them to a chemical that is solvent, safe and easily washed through urine. While EDTA to some extent also flushes out beneficial compounds and elements, such as zinc and Vitamin B-6, these beneficial substances are replaced during the chelating process. A mixture of EDTA and vitamins and minerals is placed in an intravenous solution, and the patient takes an intravenous drip in a clinic's outpatient room. The patient usually sits beside others who watch television or read or simply visit with one another.

According to physicians who routinely use Chelation Therapy with their patients, it takes about 20 to 22 treatments for first results to make themselves known to the patient. Depending on severity of the patient's overall problems, s/he may need 30, 40,....., 100 treatments given, usually, at the rate of about three per week which, according to some physicians, is an optimum frequency of treatment. Other physicians may vary the frequency of treatment, depending upon the patient's condition. Evaluation of the patient should be made at 3, 6 and 12 month intervals[9].

For the treatment to be maximally effective, good dietary habits and appropriate exercise are important. Alcohol, drugs (including many prescription drugs) and smoking will reverse the whole process, again causing free-radical damage that leads to atherosclerosis and subsequent disease problems that occur as a secondary condition of the inability of cells to receive their proper nourishment. Physicians who provide patients with EDTA Chelation Therapy will also counsel on the negative effects of bad diet and consumption of alcohol, drugs and smoking. They will advise appropriate diets that will either assist in the chelating process or will, by themselves, provide the body with natural chelating mechanisms.

EDTA should not be used during pregnancy[9].

Chelation Therapy should normally be postponed until active liver diseases are properly treated or resolved, unless there is no other choice available[9].

Usually a physician will supplement EDTA treatment with proper diet counseling and antioxidants which are synergistic with the benefits of EDTA. These are Vitamins C, E, beta carotene, selenium, glutathione and a spectrum of B complex vitamins. Iron and copper are free radical catalysts and excesses may counteract the benefits of chelation therapy[9].

EDTA Safety

Any drug can be dangerous under the right conditions, to the wrong person. Even milk can be exceptionally dangerous to one who is allergic to it. According to the manner in which drug safety is determined EDTA is about 3-1/2 times safer or less toxic than taking aspirin[6]. This measure is taken from a standard known as the LD-50, the Lethal Dosage at which 50% of experimental animals will die in a specified period. "More than 500,000 patients have been treated in the United States alone, without a single reported incident of renal failure or death since 1960[43]."

As with any treatment, EDTA can be misused by those who do not follow a proper treatment protocol, and it is recommended that physicians use the protocol developed by The American College of Advancement in Medicine[7]. This pioneer organization has long sought to establish certification and standards of practices including appropriate training and education for all those physicians who wish to chelate patients.

What Conditions Are Benefited?

Some time after John Parks Trowbridge, Sr. retired from the U.S. Air Force, at age 70, it was discovered that he had an aortic aneurysm, a balloon-like swelling in the wall of the main artery. As this condition indicates a weakened structure that is likely to break and lead to quick death, he consulted with several physicians, including his son, John Parks Trowbridge, Jr., M.D. who, along with other physicians, recommended immediate surgery, which was accomplished. It was not until several years passed that the younger Trowbridge came to understand the benefits of Chelation Therapy, learning first from Robert Haskell, M.D., who told him, "Of all the regimens you can use to help your patients combat degenerative disease and restore their health, chelation therapy is the most powerful. It produces the greatest number of benefits to the body -- far beyond those of improved blood flow. If you want to get your prescribed nutrition to those parts of the body in which they must work, John, chelation therapy is the way to do it[39]."

The primary reason for recommending Chelation Therapy to you when you have degenerative disease or have aged has to do with its ability to restore your vital functions. Virtually everyone has some degree of clogging up of the 100,000 miles of plumbing. Often the process of atherosclerosis begins in children's arteries and progresses through adulthood, so that even the finest physical specimens show evidence of this beginning on autopsy. It is virtually certain that you have some of this clogging, to some degree, and that it contributes to your state of health at least indirectly.

EDTA intravenous Chelation Therapy has proved to be safe and effective in the treatment of many varied disease conditions related to abnormal or diseased vascular conditions. Because this therapy involves the vascular system, and because blood flow affects every cell in the body, it is not surprising to find a wide ranging set of lack-of-health conditions improved or outright cured after its use. According to James J. Julian, M.D.[2] EDTA Chelation Therapy reduces "toxic metal deposits, abnormal calcium deposits, blood cholesterol, blood pressure, leg cramps, pigmentation, varicosities, size of kidney stones. [It] improves circulation, skin texture and tone, vision, hearing, liver function. [It] relieves to various degrees: digitalis toxicity, lead toxicity, symptoms of senility, pain, symptoms of irregular rhythm, hypoglycemia, phlebitis, scleroderma, skin ulcers, and Wilson's Disease," a disease of the liver thought to be related to copper.

Doctor's who use Chelation Therapy would agree with James Julian. Morton Walker D.P.M. quotes Rudolph Alsleben, M.D. and Wilfrid E. Shute, M.D.[5] who have asserted that beneficial effects are: "prevents the deposit of cholesterol in the liver, reduces blood cholesterol levels, causes high blood pressure to drop in 60 percent of the cases, reverses the toxic effects of digitalis excess, converts to normal 50 percent of cardiac arrhythmias, reduces or relaxes excessive heart contractions, increases intracellular potassium, reduces heart irritability, increases the removal of lead, removes calcium from atherosclerotic plaques, dissolves kidney stones, reduces serum iron, protects against iron poisoning and iron storage disease, reduces heart valve calcification, improves heart function, detoxifies several snake and spider venoms, reduces the dark pigmentation of varicose veins, heals calcified necrotic ulcers, reduces the disabling effects of intermittent claudication, improves vision in diabetic retinopathy, decreases macular degeneration, and dissolves small cataracts."

William J. Mauer, D.O., according to Walker[5], also provided an additional listing gathered from his own and the experience of other physicians. These include: "Eliminates heavy metal toxicity, makes arterial walls more flexible, manages excess quantities of fat in the blood, prevents osteoarthritis, causes rheumatoid arthritis symptoms to disappear, has an antiaging effect, smooths skin wrinkles, offers psychological relief, assures the presence of adequate zinc in the blood, lowers insulin requirements for diabetics, and dissolves large and small thrombi."

Other physicians have listed other health improvements, including reversal of impotence, when impotence is caused by blockage or decreased flow of blood.

Chelation Therapy References

1. American College of Advancement in Medicine (ACAM), 23121 Verdugo Dr., Suite 204, Laguna Hills, CA 92653.

2. James J. Julian, M.D. ,*Chelation Extends Life*, Wellness Press, 1654 Cahuenga Boulevard, Hollywood, CA 90028, p. 31, 1982.

3. Baron, John M. D.O. personal interview and unpublished documents.

4. Personal knowledge.

5. Morton Walker, D.P.M., (Gary Gordon, M.D., Consultant) The *Chelation Answer*, M.Evans and Company, Inc., p. 18, 1982.

6. Morton Walker, D.P.M., (Gary Gordon, M.D., Consultant)*The Chelation Answer*, M.Evans and Company, Inc., p. 97, 1982.

7. di Fabio, Anthony, The *Art of Getting Well*, , The Arthritis Trust of America, 7111 Sweetgum Drive SW, Fairview, TN 37062-9384, p. 83, 1988; also see Kindle or Nook.

8. *Handbook of Chemistry and Physics*, 26th Edition, p. 1637, viscosity formula 1942;

9. *Protocol for the Safe and Effective Administration of Intravenous EDTA Chelation Therapy*, obtained from

66

one of the semiannual meetings of the American College of Advancement in Medicine (ACAM) 23121 Verdugo Dr., Suite 204, Laguna Hills, CA 92653.

10. Halstead, Bruce, The *Scientific Basis of EDTA Chelation Therapy*, Golden Quill Publishers, Inc., 1979.

11. Farr, Charles H., M.D., PhD, White, Robert L. P.A.C., PhS., Schachter, Michael, M.D., Chronological *History of EDTA Chelation Therapy*, Revised October 1991.

12. Butterfield, J.B, "Free Radical Pathology and it's Involvement in Chronic Disease Processes", *Stroke* 9: 443-445.

13. Cranton, E.M., Frackleton, J.P., "Free Radical Pathology in Age-Associated Diseases", *Journal of Holistic Medicine* 6:1.

14. Collin, Jonathan, M.D., "Free Radical Pathology and Chelation Therapy", *Townsend Letter for Doctors.* 1984.

15. Carter, James P., Olszewer, Efrain, "EDTA Chelation Therapy in Chronic Degenerative Disease", *Medical Hypotheses* (1988) 27: 41-49.

16. Evers, Ray, M.D., "Chemo-Endarterectory Therapy and Preventive Medicine", *Townsend Letter for Doctors*, Feb/Mr. 1986. Issue #49.

17. Josephson, Emanuel M., M.D., "Glaucoma and Its Medical Treatment With Cortin," *JAQA*, Vol. 3, No. 1, p. 2-6, Oct. 1987.

18. Morton Walker, D.P.M., (Gary Gordon, M.D., Consultant)*The Chelation Answer*, M.Evans and Company, Inc., p.113, 1982.

19. Morton Walker, D.P.M., (Gary Gordon, M.D., Consultant)*The Chelation Answer*, M.Evans and Company, Inc., p.175, 1982. Quoting from Jane E. Brody, "Doctors query bypass surgery as aid to heart." *New York Times*, November 22, 1976.

20. Lau, Benjamin, M.D., Ph.D., *Garlic Research Update*, Odyssey Publishing, Inc. 2135 West 45th Avenue, Vancouver, B.C., Canada V6M 2J2, p.2-3, 1991.

21. Personal Conversation with George Klabin.

22. Elmer Cranton, Ed., *A Textbook on EDTA Chelation Therapy, Special Issue of Journal of Advancement in Medicine*, Volume 2, Numbers 1/2, Human Sciences Press, Inc, 233 Spring Street, New York, New York 10013-1578, p. 18, Spring/Summer 1989.

23. Zigurts Strauts, M.D., *Townsend Letter for Doctors*, p. 382-383, May 1992.

24. Elmer Cranton, Ed., *A Textbook on EDTA Chelation Therapy, Special Issue of Journal of Advancement in Medicine*, Volume 2, Numbers 1/2, Human Sciences Press, Inc, 233 Spring Street, New York, New York 10013-1578, p. 34, Spring/Summer 1989 .

25. Elmer Cranton, Ed., *A Textbook on EDTA Chelation Therapy, Special Issue of Journal of Advancement in Medicine*, Volume 2, Numbers 1/2, Human Sciences Press, Inc, 233 Spring Street, New York, New York 10013-1578, p. 36, Spring/Summer 1989 .

26. Arabinda Das, "Complementary medical Treatment for Coronary Heart Disease," *Townsend Letter for Doctors*, p. 419, May 1992.

27. H. Richard Casdorph, M.E., Ph.D. "EDTA Chelation Therapy: Efficacy in Arteriorslerotic Heart Disease," Elmer Cranton, Ed., *A Textbook on EDTA Chelation Therapy, Special Issue of Journal of Advancement in Medicine*, Volume 2, Numbers 1/2, Human Sciences Press, Inc, 233 Spring Street, New York, New York 10013-1578, p. 121, Spring/Summer 1989.

28. H. Richard Casdorph, M.E., Ph.D. "EDTA Chelation Therapy: Efficacy in Arteriorslerotic Heart Disease," Elmer Cranton, Ed., *A Textbook on EDTA Chelation Therapy, Special Issue of Journal of Advancement in*

68

Medicine, Volume 2, Numbers 1/2, Human Sciences Press, Inc, 233 Spring Street, New York, New York 10013-1578, p. 131, Spring/Summer 1989.

29. E.W. McDonagh, D.O., FACGP, C.J. Rudolph, D.O., Ph.D., and E. Cheraskin, M.D., D.M.D. "An Oculo-cerebrovasculometric Analysis of the Improvement in Arterial Stenosis Following EDTA Chelation Therapy," Elmer Cranton, Ed., *A Textbook on EDTA Chelation Therapy, Special Issue of Journal of Advancement in Medicine,* Volume 2, Numbers 1/2, Human Sciences Press, Inc, 233 Spring Street, New York, New York 10013-1578, p. 155, Spring/Summer 1989.

30. E.W. McDonagh, D.O., FACGP, C.J. Rudolph, D.O., Ph.D., and E. Cheraskin, M.D., D.M.D. "Effect of EDTA Chelation Therapy Plus Multivitamin Trace Mineral Supplementation Upon Vascular Dynamics: Ankle/ Brachial Doppler Systolic Blood Pressure Ratio, "Elmer Cranton, Ed., *A Textbook on EDTA Chelation Therapy, Special Issue of Journal of Advancement in Medicine,* Volume 2, Numbers 1/2, Human Sciences Press, Inc, 233 Spring Street, New York, New York 10013-1578, p. 159, Spring/Summer 1989.

31. H. Richard Casdorph, M.D., Ph.D. and Charles H. Farr, M.D., Ph.D. "EDTA Chelation Therapy: Treatment of Peripheral Arterial Occlusion, an Alternative to Amputation," Elmer Cranton, Ed., *A Textbook on EDTA Chelation Therapy, Special Issue of Journal of Advancement in Medicine,* Volume 2, Numbers 1/2, Human Sciences Press, Inc, 233 Spring Street, New York, New York 10013-1578, p. 167, Spring/Summer 1989.

32. Walter Blumer, M.D., and H. Richard Casdorph, M.D., Ph.D. "Ninety Percent Reduction in Cancer Mortality After Chelation therapy With EDTA," Elmer Cranton, Ed., *A Textbook on EDTA Chelation Therapy, Special Issue of Journal of Advancement in Medicine,* Volume 2,

Numbers 1/2, Human Sciences Press, Inc, 233 Spring Street, New York, New York 10013-1578, p. 183, Spring/Summer 1989.

33. Efrain Olszewer, M.D. and James P. Carter, M.D., Dr. PH, "EDTA Chelation Therapy: A Retrospective Study of 2,870 Patients," Elmer Cranton, Ed., *A Textbook on EDTA Chelation Therapy, Special Issue of Journal of Advancement in Medicine*, Volume 2, Numbers 1/2, Human Sciences Press, Inc, 233 Spring Street, New York, New York 10013-1578, p. 197, Spring/Summer 1989.

34. American Heart Association, *Heart and Stroke Facts*, 1992.

35. Personal Communication from Warren Levin, M.D.

36. E.L. Hannan, H. Kilburn, Jr., H. Bernard, J.F. O'Donnell, G. Lukacik, E.P. Shields, "Coronary Artery Bypass surgery: The Relationship Between Inhospital Mortality Rate and Surgical Volume After Controlling for Clinical Risk Factors, *Med-Care*, Nov 1991, 29(11): 1094-107.

37. G.T. O'Connor, S.K. Plume, E.M. Olmstead, L.H. Coffin, J.R. Morton, C.T. Maloney, E.R. Nowicki, J.F. Tryzelaar, F. Hernandez, L. Adrian, et. al. "A Regional Prospective Study of In-Hospital Mortality Associated with Coronary Artery Bypass Grafting, *"JAMA*, Aug 14, 1991, 266(6): 803-9.

38. J. Zelen, T.V. Bilfinger, C.E. Anagnostopoulos, Coronary Artery Bypass Grafting. The relationship of Surgical Volume, Hospital Location, and Outcome, *NY State J Med*, Jul 1991 91(7): 290-2.

39. John Parks Trowbridge, M.D., Morton Walker, D.P.M., *The Healing Powers of Chelation Therapy*, New Way of Life, Inc., 484 High Ridge Road, Stamford, CT 06905, 1991.

40. *Chelation Therapy*, Morton Walker, D.P.M.

Freelance Communications, 484 High Ridge Road, Stamford,Ct 06905, 1980.

41. *The Chelation Way*, Morton Walker, D.P.M. Avery Publishing Group, Inc., Garden City Park, New York,1990.

42. "Radical Concerns Over Drinking Water," *Science News*, Vol. 141, No. 24, June 13, 1992, p. 398.

43. Efrain Olszewer, M.D., Fuad Calil Sabbag, M.D., and James P. Carter, M.D., Dr. PH., "A Pilot Double-Blind Study of Sodium-Magnesium EDTA in Peripheral Vascular Disease," *Journal of the National Medical Association*, Vol. 82, No.3, March 1990.

44. James P. Frackelton, M.D., "Letters to the Editors," *Townsend Letter for Doctors*, July 1992.

45. James P. Frackelton, M.D., "Letters to the Editors," *Townsend Letters for Doctors*, p. 604, July 1992.

46. Gordon E. Potter, M.D. "The Blood/Brain Connection,' *Townsend Letter for Doctors*, July 1992.

47. Personal Communication from Warren Levin, M.D. to Perry A. Chapdelaine, Sr.

Recommended Readings on Chelation Therapy

1. Elmer Cranton, Ed., *A Textbook on EDTA Chelation Therapy, Special Issue of Journal of Advancement in Medicine*, Volume 2, Numbers 1/2, Human Sciences Press, Inc, 233 Spring Street, New York, New York 10013-1578, Spring/Summer, 1989.

2. di Fabio, Anthony, *The Art of Getting Well*, The Arthritis Trust of America, 7111 Sweetgum Drive SW, Fairview, TN 37062-9384, 1988; Also on Kindle or Nook.

3. Morton Walker, D.P.M., (Gary Gordon, M.D., Consultant)*The Chelation Answer*, M.Evans and Company, Inc., 1982.

4. Halstead, Bruce, *The Scientific Basis of EDTA Chelation Therapy*, Golden Quill Publishers, Inc., 1979.

5. James J. Julian, M.D. ,*Chelation Extends Life*, Wellness Press, 1654 Cahuenga Boulevard, Hollywood,

CA 90028, 1982.

6. *Protocol for the Safe and Effective Administration of Intravenous EDTA Chelation Therapy*, obtained from one of the semiannual meetings of the American College of Advancement in Medicine (ACAM) 23121 Verdugo Dr., Suite 204, Laguna Hills, CA 92653.

7. John Parks Trowbridge, M.D., Morton Walker, D.P.M., *The Healing Powers of Chelation Therapy*, New Way of Life, Inc., 484 High Ridge Road, Stamford, CT 06905.

8. *Townsend Letter for Doctors*, 911 Tyler Street, Port Townsend, WA 98368-6541.

9. Roy Kupsinel, M.D, Ed., *Health Consciousness*, ., PO Box 550, Oviedo, FL 32765.

10. Morton Walker, D.P.M., *Chelation Therapy*, Freelance Communications, 484 High Ridge Road, Stamford,Ct 06905, 1980.

11. Morton Walker, D.P.M., *The Chelation Way*, Avery Publishing Group, Inc., Garden City Park, New York,1990.

Stress Management

Stress Management is absolutely essential for the Rheumatoid Arthritic. The reason is this: When we are under stress, adrenaline is produced which turns on cortisone in the form of a substance called "cortisol." Cortisol, to provide us with quick energy during emergencies, causes small proteins in the immunological system to be utilized as a quick energy source. When we are under stress continually, this process goes on continually. The utilization of portions of the immunological system as quick energy causes the natural balance of cells responsible for defending us from invaders to be upset, and that, in effect, creates a kind of weakening of the immunological system. The weakening of the immunological system permits organisms of opportunity (such as the yeast/

fungus *Candidas albicans*) to spread throughout the body, which further creates problems[3].

How Can Rheumatoid Arthritis Be Treated?

Rheumatoid Arthritis is known as "the great crippler," and as such, this condition frightens a great many. Established medical doctrine does not admit to any solution or knowledge on how to make one so afflicted well. According to *Clinics in Rheumatic Diseases*[11], a peer-reviewed summary of peer-reviewed research literature, established treatments are statistically no more effective than if the afflicted were left alone, or about one out of three would spontaneously remit; i.e, be "improved" — at least for the moment — if left alone. Actually the statistics are somewhat worse when one realizes that traditional immuno-modulating drugs such as methotrexate (or other cytotoxic drugs), cyclosporin, gold, penicillamine and long-term corticosteroids are not only <u>not</u> effective but also further damage the immunological system. It is hardly recommended, therefore, that any kind of traditional treatments including the above damaging drugs be accepted by one suffering from Rheumatoid Disease.

<u>General Rules to Wellness</u>

As already described, one must search out and remove (or remove self from) causation of stress[2].

Second, as already described, nutritional guidance and vitamin and mineral and essential fatty acid supplements must be sought[21].

A whole life-style change may be involved in accepting the two recommendations above, and so the question the afflicted must ask is this: Do I want to be well strongly enough to affect changes of life-style and diet? Or will I continue to raise barriers against wellness by finding reasons why I can't change my life-style and diet?

Third, a holistically oriented physician will begin to rule out other conditions that the body uses to mimic

Rheumatoid Arthritis. These may include, but not be limited to, external allergies from various pollutants and known allergens, internal allergies such as from food, air or drink, Candidiasis, bacterial pathogens (from ticks: Lyme Disease, for example), and from the inability to properly bring nourishment through the blood stream because of atherosclerosis. In this latter condition, of course, would be recommended Chelation Therapy[2].

Fourth, a holistically oriented physician may also want to determine if the hormonal system is in balance and, if replacement hormones are suggested, to so provide them to the patient[6].

Fifth, you and the holistically oriented physician together must determine any other treatments required for you.

Sixth, do not believe that there is no hope, no cure, just because a particular treatment has not worked, or because a particular doctor knows too little to help you.

Seventh, keep trying! Most folks get well rapidly once they take charge of their own lives, assume responsibility for all that has happened to them, and begin to learn how to reverse their ills.

Allergies and Weakened Immunological System

Of all the conditions that create symptoms perceivable as "arthritic" certain ones seem to be most prominent. Candidias and others will be discussed briefly.

Candidiasis[41,42,43,71]

The yeast/fungus *Candidas albicans*, is an ever-present microorganism. C. Orian Truss, M.D. first identified the characteristics and symptomatic patterns that deduced whether or not an individual was being overwhelmed by this organism. *Candidas albicans* invades various parts of bodily tissues, resulting in localized infections. Common sites of infection are the mouth as in infant Thrush, gastrointestinal tract, vagina, urinary tract, prostate gland, skin, fingernails and toenails. Under normal conditions your body is able to resist this invasion, as it does other germs. Whenever various substances weaken the immunological system, the yeast/fungus begins to spread, and creates havoc throughout body parts and systems. It may cripple the immune system so that it can no longer repel invaders. It can create allergies to chemicals and foods. It is believed that it invades the intestinal wall where toxins from microorganisms and protein molecules from food enter the blood stream directly from the intestinal tract. Once inside the bloodstream these foreign proteins are recognized as foreign antigens and the body manufactures antibodies to it. This is the start of additional food allergies which progresses with the progress of Rheumatoid Disease[2].

Treatment for Candidiasis has a clear relationship to bringing about wellness in the Rheumatoid Disease patient as well as having a strong contribution to the general subject of allergies.

Other Allergies

Allergies are often described as being extrinsic (to the body) or intrinsic. Examples of extrinsic are pollen, chemicals (actually chemical sensitivities, not allergies), fabrics, and so on. Examples of intrinsic are: (1) foreign invaders protozoa, bacteria, mycoplasma, yeast/fungus, virus or toxins produced by these microorganisms; and (2) residual chemicals or derivatives of chemicals that are stored in lipids (fatty parts) in the cells. Intolerance to foods may be genetically derived or might very well be from weakened intestinal lining from such agents as Candidiasis.

As any of the above allergies (or chemical sensitivities) can (1) produce symptoms that mimic various arthritic symptoms and (2) contribute to free radical pathology that enforces the arthritic condition, serious attention should be paid to either avoidance of the allergenic sub-stances or treatments that cure the underlying allergenic response.

Treatments for Extrinsic and Intrinsic Allergies

There are various alternative treatments reported to have affect on the course of otherwise intransigent aller-gies. These are Ozone Therapy[32,35] Photopheresis, Hydrogen Peroxide (IV) Therapy[31,34,35,37,39] Car-nivora Pitcher Plant (Venus Fly Trap) Therapy[44], Euro-pean Live Cell Therapy[85], and Bee Pollen[30,45, 46,55,81]. No one is entirely sure how all of these treat-ments function, but they obviously have an underlying ability to strengthen the immunological system, provide proper nourishment and/or enzymes, or help in the repair of crucial organs. J.O. Hunter found that food intolerance has been implicated in many conditions, and exclusion diets were found to be effective when treating "migraine, Crohn's disease, eczema, hyperactivity and rheumatoid arthritis[80]." Additional treatments include Bio-Detoxi-fication and Clinical Ecological Treatment.

Bio-Detoxification

Bio-Detoxification covers a broad spectrum of vari-ous means for ridding the body of undesirable pollutants found in either the intestinal tract or the fatty parts of cells (lipids.) According to Jeffrey S. Bland, Ph.D., J.O. Hunter points to abnormal bacterial flora in patients with rheuma-toid arthritis and ankylosing spondylitis, as well as Crohn's disease[80]. Hunter concluded that "if food allergy is not an immunological disease in many patients, it may rather be a disorder of bacterial fermentation in the colon and might appropriately be named an `enterometabolic disor-der' associated with metabolic toxicity[80]." Colon cleans-ers are widely used to remove pathogens and long-stand-ing feces from the colon, where pathogens live. Others address the whole intestinal tract by means of various drugs, herbs, and/or other substances such as fatty acids inimical to *Candidas albicans* and other pathogens. They will use products intended to scrape out these organisms, or a combination of removal and killing of the pathogenic organisms such as combinations of Psyllium seed with Bentonite and Capyrillic/Virgin Olive Oils. There is also simultaneous replacement with natural microflora: *Lactobacillus acidophilus* and *Bifido bacteria*[56].

Clinical Ecology

Clinical Ecology[2,47] addresses itself primarily to determining the specific nature of the allergen and then laying out a course of action for avoiding it. Theron Randolph, M.D. is considered the grandaddy of this approach which has found numerous successful practitioners. Quite surprisingly, at least to the layman, Theron Randolph's work and the work of other physicians such as Marshall Mandell, M.D. (Alan Mandell Clinic) has clearly shown that addictions to particular foods are based upon an allergy reaction and, in that sense at least, food allergies and their addictions have a physiological similarity to drug addictions. A chocolateholic, for example, is almost surely allergic to chocolate. Those foods we purchase most frequently, and <u>really like</u> , are often the chief source of allergic reactions. Theron Randolph, M.D., Marshall Mandell, M.D. and many other physicians have shown that people may become allergic to almost anything. One person, for example, was known to be allergic to tantalum sutures[52], a substance originally chosen as one that was non-allergenic. Others have found themselves allergic to every kind of food, natural and automobile gas and oil, any kind of fabrics, air and water pollutants and food preservatives and contaminants, and so on. By isolating the individual in a clinic constructed to be allergy free, and then by exhausting the intestinal tract through a five day fast, with nothing except pure water to drink, the individual can find their specific allergens. Usually, after the fast, this is done by trying one food at a time. When a substance is ingested that has allergenic properties, the individual usually has a more severe reaction than before this trial. When one learns all of the possible allergens, and returns to normal life, s/he must be most careful about exposure to these substances, either eliminating them as food or from the environment completely, or taking them as foods but sparingly, usually only once every third or so day[2,47].

Sauna Bio-Detoxification

Zane Gard, M.D. and Erma J. Brown, B.S.N., Ph.N. state that "According to the EPA, by 1980 over 400 chemicals had been detected in human tissue; 48 were found in adipose tissue, 40 in breastmilk, 73 in liver, and over 250 in blood. The National Academy of Sciences reports that an average American today ingests about 40 mg of pesticides each day as DDT, each year in food sources alone -- and carries approximately 1/10th of a gram permanently stored in body fat. "Human accumulation of such compounds as DDT, PCP, PCB, THC, and dioxin, reflect biologically persistent chemicals which are partitioned within the body from water into lipids. . . . "Chemicals stored in the body pose a serious threat to both physiological and psychological health. . . . the human body has no previous experience with these chemicals and there is no natural machinery in the body to break them down, much less eliminate them.[82]."

None of the previously described treatments will totally eliminate pollutants stored in the fatty parts of each cell (lipids). One method that has proven to be quite effective is that of proper use of sweat saunas coupled with the proper mixture of replacement water, vitamins, minerals and essential fatty acids and exercise. This detoxification is known by several names, among which are those of Sauna Bio-detoxification and The Purification Rundown®.

Although sweat saunas have been used for centuries, the first to take up a systematic study of biological and psychological phenomena that saunas produce is that of L. Ron Hubbard, founder of the philosophy of The Church of Scientology[2,48].

One of the first scientific studies of Hubbard's development and hypothesis -- that residual pollutants stored in the fatty parts of cells were the triggering agents for many diseases and misunderstood psychological phenomena -- was funded by the United States Environmental Protection Agency and conducted by David W. Schnare, Max Ben, and Megan G. Shields, M.D.[2. 49]. Their study showed that PCBs and PBBs and Chlorinated Pesticides were reduced considerably through the use of Hubbard's regimen. Later studies[2,50,51,82] have verified this finding, and have extended the range of detoxified elements to include many otherwise intransigents, including so-called recreational drugs and medicines that have similar adverse affects.

Besides the aforementioned vitamins and minerals and essential fatty acids and replacement water, the patient is exposed to 140 degrees F to 180 degrees F for 3-1/2 to 4-1/2 hours each day, also being permitted to leave the sauna and shower or walk around, and to eat, from time to time. In a clinical setting, tests are made of residual poisons in the lipids; in the Hubbard detoxification setting, another person familiar with the routine takes the sauna with you. Easily observed phenomena determines whether or not the replacement vitamins, minerals and essential fatty acids will be increased at each session. The person undergoing this sauna will subjectively feel that s/he is reliving portions of past experiences where s/he was exposed to the substances that produced the residual chemicals now stored in the fatty parts of cells. For example, one person[52] felt like he was again being treated with chloroform during an operation (smell, taste, other sensations), and then later experienced nitrous oxide gas from a former dental extraction. Many people experience suntan exposures, their skin showing vivid marks of bathing suit straps and the suit itself.

According to Zane R. Gard, M.D. and Erma J. Brown, B.S.N, Ph.N. "Medical conditions reported to have shown improvement on the program include the following: myopia, bursitis/fibromyositis, irritable bowel, dermatitis, acne, dysmenorrhea, tension headaches, hypoglycemia, fluid retention, thyromegaly, migraine headaches, allergic rhinitis, seborrhea, hypertension, pyorrhea, paraplegia, Peyronies Disease, and Grave's Disease[82]." They also observed "improvement in [a] large array of unrelated medical conditions[82]."

Unfortunately there are very few clinics established to furnish this method, but fortunately The Church of Scientology[R] has forged ahead to make the process available everywhere in the world[2].

Dental (Mercury)Toxicity

Mercury Toxicity probably produces more symptoms of various debilitating disease than any other substance, because the use of Mercury in teeth as dental fillings is and has been so widespread, and its medical implications so little understood by either the American Medical Association (until recently) or the American Dental Association. The Swedish Dental Association, after many years of resistance, finally accepted the multitude of scientific evidence that exists, and apologized to the Swedish public for the Dental Association's prior intransigence.

Briefly, according to the FDA and researchers, there is no lower limit to a safe exposure to mercury, and as fillings are composed of mercury, silver, copper, tin and zinc, there are different electro-potentials in each filling. When dissimilar metals, with differing electro-potentials are bathed in acid (or alkali), a current is formed. That's how batteries produce current. As saliva is acidic (or in a healthy person, alkaline), current is produced in each filling of each tooth. This current, along with other micro-organisms and acid (or base) itself cause mercury to slowly vaporize and to combine with organic materials to be absorbed and accumulated in the body. Not only do people become exceedingly sensitive to mercury itself, but they also manifest a variety of symptoms that are often misdiagnosed as something else. One physician almost routinely rules out mercury poisoning by first asking his patients to have their fillings replaced by non-harmful ingredients, especially if electric current tests read dangerously. Mercury detoxification is an important part of ridding of allergies. Mercury poisoning may simulate symptoms of other diseases, such as Osteoarthritis and Rheumatoid Disease[54].

Energy Medicine: Electromagnetics and Bio-Magnetics

Modern medical science, with some exceptions (electricity, radiation), has been oriented toward chemical solutions to human problems. The physics of human physiology has been handily ignored, although "the fact that magnetic fields can be an aid in alleviating human suffering has been known since ancient times," according to William H. Philpott, M.D. and Dean R.Bonlie, D.D.S.[104].

ELF Laboratory's Courtland Reeves says, "Advancing the concept of magnetics is *Energy Medicine*. While magnetics uses "static" magnetic fields to influence energy patterns or charge on the physical/material particle, Energy Science uses "pulsating" fields to influence energy patterns surrounding the physical/material particle. Energy medicine recognizes that the body operates in a dynamic environment where matter is composed primarily of charged energy particles. To address physical problems, the `standard of care' should also consider the electrical and energetic charge surrounding the `damaged cell'. The Energy Science formula for health includes standard variables such as chemical imbalances, nutrition, immune system requirements, mental health, stress and other standard factors, but also includes the cell's `energetic' component as part of the `standard of care'[113]."

Even though patients follow all the best known "standard-of- care" advice, they cannot improve their health condition. "It is as though they have hit a `brick wall' and something blocks their progress to better health[113]."

"Energy [medical] scientists believe that the `standard prescription' for health should also look at the reestablishment of the fundamental `charge' or `energetic' value of the diseased cell. Energy Medicine's primary contribution to the health equation is to provide assistance in boosting the `energetic capacitance' in the biofield surrounding the diseased cell. Once the damaged cell's energetic value is stabilized or returned to normal, the cell seems to accept or process more quickly, the many benefits provided by `standard prescription' care[113]."

With the development of sensitive magnetometers, i.e. squid, evidence of the presence of magnetic fields at the cellular level is easily witnessed[104.

The importance of this cellular electromagnetic field is beginning to emerge, and many physicians are using this new knowledge for both diagnosis and treatment. Apparently a positive electromagnetic field is a polarity associated with injury, whereas a negative electromagnetic field is a polarity associated with healing[104]. This feature is so important that Robert R. Barefoot and Carl J. Reich, M.D. reported on "another major biological event ... ignored by most of the medical community. In the early 1970's, the surgeon Cynthia Illingworth of the Sheffield

Children's Hospital in England accidentally found that when a young child's finger is sheared off beyond the outermost crease of the outermost or last joint, and the wound is dressed *but not closed*, the finger will grow back perfectly within three months. By 1974 Illingworth documented the *regrowth* of several hundred fingertips[102]."

Understanding why the suturing of a severed fingertip prohibits restoration of the fingertip through normal growth functions also involves an understanding of the relationship between electromagnetic polarities induced by suturing. The production of a positive electromagnetic polarity prevents the regrowth, and positive electromagnetic polarity comes about through the traditional practice of suturing up the severed finger.

According to Elf Laboratory's Courtland Reeves, "Energy medicine uses `pulsating' fields to influence the energy patterns surrounding the diseased cell. Traditional medicine as practiced by Native Americans and ancient medical practitioners, used both `chemical' and `energetic' medicine in the `standard of care' for treating disease. These `standards of care' recognized the physical and energetic properties of the body and combined chemical (herb preparations) and `energetic (acoustical and pulsating fields) to effect healing[113]." [Native Americans or ancient cultures, used natural herbs or ingredients applied to the skin for absorption, music or rhythmic word chanting to produce acoustical wave forms to interact with bioenergy fields, hand held devices (i.e., a gourd or stick with feathers) that initiated a static field which is shaken to oscillate at a specific rhythmic frequency to produce a frequency pattern which also interacts with biofield energy.]

"Research by Becker has shown that bioenergy fields have a functional role when he measured the `current of injury' associated with wounds and bone fractures[114].

Additional evidence supports the conclusion that locally generated endogenous energy fields mediate the natural healing process. Intrinsic fields of the body are now known to be generated during various healthy and diseased states: (1) periods of rapid cell division (either during natural growth processes like skin cell growth or during abnormal cell growth associated with hyperprolific diseases like cancer; (2) intense nervous activity associated with mental processes or thoughts; or (3) various pathological conditions like those associated with bone fracture.

"Recent evidence for the functional role of intrinsic body energy fields has shown that very weak, pulsating electromagnetic fields, similar to those generated by the body, when applied to the body, can promote healing of the body. Extremely low fields, when artificially produced, have been shown to directly affect a wide variety of tissues including the immune system, the cardiovascular system and the muscular-skeletal system[115]. These biological effects have now been confirmed in laboratories throughout the world and demonstrated at the clinical, animal and cellular level.

"In rheumatoid disease, physical symptoms often include swelling, tenderness and calcium deposits at the site of injury. Energy medicine researchers note the one condition underlying most pain is swollen tissue. Analyzing electrical characteristics of the principal material in tissue, researchers find protein interactions (bondings) are priorily electrical. When a protein molecule becomes `destabilized' or `loses a charged particle' it becomes a `free radical' and must couple with another molecule to correct its `out of balance' condition. Protein molecules' stability is reestablished when it couples with the H_2O molecule. When this coupling occurs, this condition leads to water retention; swelling in interstitium of the connective tissue;

blockages in the lymphatic system; buildup of toxic waste material; and swelling, severe oedema or pain.

"Energy medicine strives to correct the cell's `out of balance' condition by producing an environment which provides reestablishment of the correct charge to the destabilized cell. Recent advances in technology have resulted in the development of a non-invasive instrument, called the Light Beam Generator™ (LBG). The LBG (using cold gas ionization) addresses the underlying cause of most pain and swelling -- a blocked lymphatic system. When the lymph fluid backs up because of blockage, pressure builds up in the lymph capillary, in the cell bed, resulting in the whole system becoming toxic due to waste disposal failure. This toxicity prevents the cells from getting necessary nutrients. Under these conditions, the cells lose metabolic efficiency and fail to do their assigned job. If enough cells are in this state, degenerative conditions are free to develop or fail to respond to treatments.

"Using cold gas ionization, lymphatic congestion and blockages are charged with incoherent light, creating an environment allowing molecules to repel each other. Therefore, trapped blood protein clusters are broken up and unobstructed lymphatic flow is reestablished. Clearing the lymph system, a component of the immune system, significantly enhances the efficiency of the body to deal with pathological conditions. Cold gas ionization lymphatic therapy [coupled with Voder Lymph Massage] enhances healing primarily through the action of the immune system's anti-infective lymph system, in combination with other `standard of care' treatment procedures, the body's natural healing abilities can be greatly enhanced. The LBG's non-invasive technique, supplies the missing `energetic' variable to the traditional `standard of care' health equation. Energy medicine researchers believe, that by adding this variable, it helps condition the cell `energetically' and accelerates the cell's ability to accept and process benefits provided from the traditional `standard of care' for rheumatoid disease treatment.

"For rheumatoid pain treatment, the LBG created environment, promotes protein clusters to separate to produce a state of free flow providing immediate reduction in swelling and tenderness. This reduction in swelling and pain is often permanent -- providing the subject continues with the acceptable `standard of care' for treatment of the rheumatoid condition[113]." ["Standard-of-care" shouldn't mean methotrexate, gold, penicillamine, long term corticosteroid, and the like, all of which will damage the patient further.]

"Electromagnetics is of equal importance to human health and happiness as biochemistry. However, there is currently throughout the world a marked surge of the application of static magnetics to both the practice of medicine and the self-help use of magnetics[104]." There is a great deal of confusion between the use of magnets and the use of electromagnetic fields. The usage of magnets has many pitfalls, not the least of which is the fact that the earth's magnetic field is about .05 gauss, whereas some static magnets are 2-6,000 gauss, and will clearly create more problems of sickness than is being addressed, chiefly by permanently or semi-permanently fouling up the body's natural electromagnetic fields. There are other problems with the usage of static magnets described in Ilanka Harezi's article, "The Danger of the Magnet Buzz," that the wary potential user should review before making a decision.

There is growing evidence that many of the electromagnetic fields and biomagnetic fields surrounding us at work and in the home affect our health adversely. If these fields truly affect us, then the haphazard usage of similar fields can also possibly harm us. If electromagnetics and biomagnetics can help us toward wellness when properly applied, it's reasonable to assume that it can also harm us when used wrongly. Unfortunately, all of the evidence is not in for either side of the question as yet, but the field of electromagnetics warrants your serious investigation and concerns.

The Arthritis fund/The Rheumatoid Disease Foundation Recommendations

The nonprofit The Arthritis Trust of America/The Rheumatoid Disease Foundation has a four-part treatment recommendation that has been very effective with many for the past ten years. They recommend that (1) certain prescription medications be given to kill off assumed internal pathogens (bacteria, protozoa, mycoplasmas, virus, yeast/fungus) to which an individual exhibits genetic susceptibility, (2) nutrition be changed so that bodily tissues become alkaline as measured by the litmus saliva test[102], (3) interneural injections be given to dampen the pain at the joints, especially while enduring a Herxheimer effect from number (1) above, and (4) other treatments such as for Candidiasis, Chelation Therapy, Allergies, hormonal replacement therapy, Reconstructive and Neural Therapy and so on as the patient requires[1,2].

Medicines used for the treatment and remission or cure of Rheumatoid Disease (Arthritis) and related collagen diseases are the following: 1. Metronidazole, 2. Clotrimazole, 3. Tinidazole, 4. Nimorazole, 5. Ornidazole, 6. Allopurinol, 7. Furazolidone, 8. Diiodohydroxyquinon, 9. Rifampin, 10. Potassium Para Amino Benzoate, 11. Copper Ions. (Contributors to the above list are Roger Wyburn-Mason, M.D., Ph.D., Jack M. Blount, M.D., Robert Bingham, M.D., and Seldon Nelson, D.O.)

The first five mentioned above are classed as 5-nitroimidazoles, where the first nitrogen in a 5-ring nitrogen structure has been replaced by another radical. Any one of them is taken at the rate of 2 grams per day, two days in a row, then skip for five days, and repeat in all for six weeks. The two grams daily for 2 days in a row dosage is computed on the basis of a 170# weight, and for each 25# above or below this weight, 1/4 of a gram is added or deducted from the 2 grams, respectively.

Simultaneously with one of the above five 5-nitroimidazoles is given 300 milligrams of number (6) above, Allopurinol, 3 times a day for 7 days. If you are one of the rare individuals who is allergic to Allopurinol, then number (7) above, Furazolidone, may be substituted at the rate of 100 mg 4 times a day, for one week.

If the disease process has not been stopped, then repeat again for another 6 weeks. Any of the above 5-nitroimidazoles, or other drugs, may be used next, or even combinations of them, if the physician deems it proper.

Diiodohydroxyquinon (Iodoquinol) should be taken as 650 mg three times a day, for three weeks. Potassium Para Amino Benzoate should be taken as 2 grams 6 times daily for two weeks.

Metronidzole is available in the United States via prescription. Clotrimazole, approved for use in the United States and Canada, is available at only limited pharmacies in the United States and Canada. Tinidazole is available virtually everywhere in the world without a prescription, except in the United States. It is very low-cost in Mexico over the counter. Nimorazole and Ornidazole are available in various European countries. In addition to items (1) and (2), items (6) through (10) are all available in the United States by prescription. Allopurinol is routinely used for Gout, and so is easily available. Furazolidone is used in the Southwestern United States for certain parasitic infections. Diiodohydrooxyquinon is used against malaria. Rifampin is used against Tuberculosis -- use

Rifampin only under close medical supervision, and as a last resort. Rifampin should be taken as 600 mg daily for one month. Potassium Para Amino Benzoate is used for certain skin disturbances. The Copper Ions, invented by Seldon Nelson, D.O.[72] may be available only through restricted sources.

Three among the more than 100 Rheumatoid Diseases that may require additional forms of treatment are Psoriasis[15], Lupus Erythematosus[14], and Scleroderma[14].

In the event of Psoriasis, the recommendation is a combination of diet and fumaric acid ester.

For Lupus Erythematosus or Scleroderma, a treatment developed by Ron Davis, M.D.[14] has proved quite effective, using both metronidazole and an injectable form of EDTA (Ethylene Diamine Tetracetic Acid) with DMSO (Dimethyl Sulfoxide).

The Jarisch-Herxheimer Effect[1,2,13,99]

Understanding the Herxheimer[13,99] effect is a key to understanding many treatment processes. In 1902 research physicians, Doctors Adolph Jarisch Herxheimer and Karl Herxheimer, studied the treatment of syphilis using various kinds of relatively dangerous medicines. They learned, and concluded, that whenever an organism more complex than a simple bacterium was killed inside the human body, one had "flu-like" symptoms. This phenomena was later named the Jarisch-Herxheimer effect, or simply "The Herxheimer." It is called "The Herxheimer Effect" when treating Tuberculosis, Rheumatoid Disease, Leishmaniasis, or some other tropical diseases. When treating Leprosy it is called "Lucio's Phenomenon." When treating Candidiasis, it is called "The die-off effect."

Dr. Paul Pybus brought to forefront the fact that the severity of the Herxheimer correlates directly with the probability of achieving wellness[1,2,13,99].

Dr. Paul Pybus, a surgeon and Englishman who resided in South Africa, was the former Chief Medical Advisor for The Rheumatoid Disease Foundation.

Over thirty years ago he worked with Roger Wyburn-Mason, M.D. the man who brought us our first consistently successful treatment for otherwise crippling rheumatoid arthritis.

From early teachings by his mentor, Wyburn-Mason, Paul Pybus developed The Arthritis Trust of America's/ The Rheumatoid Disease Foundation's technique of intra-neural injections that is so successful for the pain of both Osteoarthritis and Rheumatoid Arthritis, and which may be the foundation for explaining one of the causative factors of Osteoarthritis.

It's a pity that many modern-day physicians have not been taught the Herxheimer, or, if they have, do not understand its importance when treating a number of diseases.

It is a phenomena that results when there is an intensification of the disease symptoms and often an expansion of similar symptoms to other places all of a temporary nature, after which the patient is improved or well. Often it appears to some as if they have the flu, and so is described as "the patient having flu-like symptoms." "Flu-like symptoms" is an oversimplification of what happens in varying cases and with varying patients.

In all cases of the Herxheimer, there is the appearance of a war or tussle going on inside the body akin to the antigen/antibody warfare, where the body produces fever, sweat, aching and swollen joints, diarrhea, nausea, and so on, in varying proportions with varying degrees depending upon state of metabolism, genetics, source of disturbance and so on.

It is the belief of some physician's that some prescription drugs wrongly are described to be toxic in a certain way because, on observing an Herxheimer reaction in the patient trying the new drug, the drug researchers (and others' observations during subsequent follow-on research and use of the drug) do not fully understand the Herxheimer and believe the cause is the drug's "toxicity." Even with a full understanding of the Herxheimer effect, a pharmaceutical company must follow the "rule of over-caution," to satisfy FDA requirements for the "health and safety" of the rest of us. Thus, even with knowledge of the Herxheimer effect, a physician researcher is not necessarily in a position whereby he can, or wants to, discriminate between drug toxicity and the Herxheimer effect.

It is necessary for the successful treatment of Rheumatoid Diseases, therefore, that a physician attend the patient who uses our treatment protocol, and that the physician fully comprehend the distinctions between specific drug toxicities and the Herxheimer effect, and also understand possible allergic responses. These distinctions probably can come only through the experiences of applied clinical practices.

Drugs do have toxicities of their own, but the essential importance for Rheumatoid Arthritics is to be able to discriminate between the two: Herxheimer effect and toxicity.

This is unfortunate, as it clouds otherwise desirable treatment modes, not just those recommended in our treatment protocols for arthritics. From another view-point, those who fully understand the distinction between the Herxheimer effect and drug toxicities find themselves with a guiding clinical tool that permits the physician early in the treatment regimen to determine the probability of success for a given patient.

We have learned that, generally speaking, the more severe the induced Herxheimer, the more probability of wellness — which is not to say that one who has a very light Herxheimer may not also get well.

Prior to Dr. Paul Pybus' work developing intraneural injections, it was felt that Osteoarthritis and Rheumatoid Arthritis had little in common, except that here and there folks with Rheumatoid Arthritis might also have some Osteoarthritis.

Perhaps it is still true, that the causes are indeed distinguishable.

But one very interesting set of experiences has come forth from the application of the Wyburn-Mason/Pybus Intraneural Treatment on both Rheumatoid and Osteo victims: joint pain and joint damage in both diseases seem to stem from the same source, namely a disturbance in certain key trigger points along the peripheral nervous system. The peripheral nerves are usually those nerves close to the surface of the body, and have no insulative layers — similar to an electric wire passing current without insulation — called the C fibers, or "unmyelinated" fibers[7].

It might very well be that Osteoarthritis can be halted with Pybus' intraneurals, along with good diet, including proper supplements, hormones and changes in life style. Those possibilities, along with Pybus' Intraneural injections are told elsewhere in our literature[1,2,7,13,99].

What Dr. Pybus had to say about the Herxheimer effect is so important, that we have copied his whole article, including his footnotes for those interested.

Dr. Paul K. Pybus on the Herxheimer Reaction [13,99]

(References in this chapter are found at the end of the section.)

"This [Herxheimer] reaction was first described by an Austrian dermatologist Jarisch Adolf Herxheimer[10] working in Vienna and Innsbruck in 1895 and shortly after this, confirmed by his brother Karl Herxheimer[1,2] also a dermatologist working in Frankfort.

"They were both mainly called upon to treat syphilitic lesions of skin by means of mercury and later arsenical and bismuth preparations. They both noticed that when treating these patients many of them developed signs of high fever, profuse perspiration, night sweats, nausea and vomiting. What was more they also observed that the skin lesions became larger and inflamed before settling down and healing. In addition they found that those cases that responded in this most violent manner healed the best and fastest. The patient was quite ill for 2-3 days after which the syphilitic lesions resolved.

"Jarisch Herxheimer accounted for this reaction as a toxic manifestation caused by the foreign proteins released from the dying spirocheates. Meanwhile his brother Karl described in detail the Herxheimer fever. There is first a febrile [feverish] phase with pyrexia (heat), malaise and often a sore throat. The lesions are then aggravated and the rash if present becomes more marked with tension in the regional lymph nodes being more pronounced. In addition the primary ulcer would become oedematous (swollen) and painful (the primary chancre is characterized by its painlessness). [In a letter to *The Lancet*, Feb. 12, 1977, p. 340 it is suggested that two of the three identifying features of a Herxheimer were known since the end of the 15th century when arsenical ointment was first used to treat the great pox which had just arrived in Europe from the New World: Ed.]

"During this reaction many other signs appeared, histologic changes such as transient acute inflammation in the lesion, a leucocytosis and lymphopaenia which was greatest as the pyrexia (heat) was at its zenith.

"It was suggested by another surgeon Heyman[8] that

these histologic changes indicate that the reaction was hypersensitivity phenomenon of the delayed type similar to the tuberculin hypersensitivity type of reaction.

"Theories as to Cause

1. *Herxheimer* et.al.[1,2,10] The phenomenon is caused by the release of endotoxin of spirochaetal breakdown products following treatment. These products are reacting with sensitized syphilitic tissue to produce exacerbation of the lesion.

2. *Milian.*[3] Suggested it was due to stimulation of the spirochaetes and inadequate medication.

3. *Jadassohn.*[9] Suggested that the direct effect of the antisyphilitic drug on the tissue was an entirely toxic reaction.

4. *Fleishman.*[4] Suggested this reaction was of a vascular reflex mediated by the autonomic nervous system.

"In 1943 Mahoney et. al.[5] first described Jarisch Herxheimer Reaction in syphilitic patients treated with penicillin and since then it has been observed that other chemotherapeutic agents that are effective with syphilis also produce a Herxheimer reaction.

"Moore et. al.[6] regard the reaction as all or none phenomenon but it was found that if the dose was less than 10 international units per kilogram body weight the reaction did not occur. The increase of the dose, however, did not increase the degree of the reaction. It also occurred equally in the seropositive and seronegative patient.

"Joulia et. al.[7] reported that during the Jarisch Herxheimer reaction the eosinophils decreased showing it to be an antigen antibody reaction. However, Heyman found that using antihistamines had no effect on the reaction whatosever.

"The Jarisch Herxheimer reaction occurs in other diseases treated with anitbiotics. It has been noted in:

1. Yaws treated with penicillin.

2. Vincents Angina treated with metronidazole.

3. Relapsing fever (also a spirochaetal disease) treated with tetracycline.

4. Rat bite fever (also due to a spirillum) treated with penicillin or tetracycline.

5. Leprosy where it is known as the Lucia phenomenon treated with Dapsone.

6. Brucellosis treated with chloramphenicol.

7. Glanders treated with erythromycin.

8. Anthrax treated with aureomycin.

9. Rheumatoid Disease treated with metronidazole [and other drugs: Ed.]

10. Psoriasis treated with metronidazole [and other drugs: Ed.]

11. [Systemic Lupus Erythematosus and Scleroderma treated with metronidazole and other drugs: Ed.]

"In 1972 Gudjonsson[11] investigated the Herxheimer reaction in adult seropositive and negative syphilitics and found a febrile [feverish] reaction in 60%. It could be produced with doses above 10 International units per kilogram. However, in 30% of cases no reaction occurred until as much as 600,000 I.U. per kg, were given and so it would appear that the higher doses produced a stronger reaction than the lower ones and this was at variance with the observations of Moore.

"He also noted an increase in the neutrophils and a decrease in the lymphocyte count which occurs when the temperature is greatest. The Eosinophil decreased and may be due to the degranulation of their cells as they phagacytose the breakdown products of the treponemes. This is also an observation in my own series of treated rheumatoid arthritic cases with metronidazole as the eosinophils are completely removed from the blood in most cases with a positive Herxheimer reaction.

"Effect of Prednisone on Herxheimer reaction. Here the Prednisone clearly influences the febrile [feverish] response at a daily dose of 40 mg. The leucocyte changes are not effected and so the Prednisone influences only the febrile component and not the other manifestations of the reaction. Gudjonsson concludes that the reaction is not of an allergic nature, but is caused by some leucocyte pyrogen released by phagocytosis of the treponemes.

Discussion

"If we say that Gudjonsson is correct and that the reaction is due to the release by the leucocytes of a pyrogen when something is phagocytosed, then this further suggests that the Herxheimer reaction seen when treating rheumatoid arthritis with certain drugs, is due to the phagocytosis of an infective agent. Thus, although no one apart from Stamm and Wyburn-Mason[12] have found amoebae for certain, this is strong evidence for an infective cause of the disease. An Herxheimer reaction is the one constant finding in all our search and the strength of the reaction correlates very closely to clinical improvement as shown separately by Prosch, Bingham and Pybus[13] [and now others: Ed.].

"Furthermore in my own recent series the correlation is shown to be 100% correct.

"I have also shown what would occur should these cases that I have done be analyzed on a double-blind study by someone who was not acquainted with the Herxheimer reaction.

"Herxheimer reaction is becoming the cornerstone of our present research and unless full account is taken of its occurrence any double-blind trial performed will tend to be misleading. The mere fact that it occurs will influence any such trial and would probably be more advantageous if the final assessor could be suitably blinded as to the previous occurrences of the Herxheimer reaction.

"I had sincerely hoped that this was being done at our double-blind studies. I have strongly advocated that it be done." [The Herxheimer reaction was not taken into account at our double-blind studies at Bowman Gray School of Medicine, thus causing the study to be inconclusive.]

"The symptoms of the Herxheimer can be most severe. They can discourage not only the patient, but also the doctor and anyone running a trial not knowing of these, will assume they are toxic symptoms and remove the patient from the trial [as occurred at our Bowman Gray School of Medicine study on use of Clotrimazole: Ed.]

"This also occurred in the original Guy's[18] trial when they came to the conclusion that metronidazole had no effect on rheumatoid arthritis and this lack of recognition of the Herxheimer reaction did untold damage to our cause. Not only were the numbers in the trial inadequate, only 20, but other medications were not stopped [Nonsteroidal anti-inflammatories: Ed.] Follow up was only for 6 weeks (they should have waited at least two months), strike dosage was usually inadequate either to produce an Herxheimer or clinical improvement (400 mg b.d.;) and the one case that did produce a reaction was withdrawn because of these 'side effects.'" [The Herxheimer effect: Ed.]

Recent Progress

"This year I have made an analysis of 24 cases of Rheumatoid Arthritis (RA) and this revealed many interesting facts.

"In a total of 288 metronidazole nights there were only 47 nights or 16.32% when nothing happened at all. All the rest (241 or 83.68%) showed some reaction and were divided up according to the following:

Heavy perspiration and night sweats	54
Flu-like symptoms	47
Rigors......................................	32
Fever	2
Headaches	85
Malaise	43
Diarrhea	19
Nausea	49
Vomiting.................................	8
Pain in other joints previously unaffected	79
Burning micturition	21
Bone pain	39
Itching	33
Flushing of skin and red patches	39

"These figures are all the more remarkable when one considers that in the normal person without rheumatoid disease, this dose of metronidazole produces no symptoms whatsoever.

"Thus, in our campaign in the treatment of rheumatoid disease, two points stand out markedly:

1. Metronidazole and our other recommended medicines work;

2. That a Herxheimer reaction occurs in at least 83% of metronidazole nights.

"These two points seem to prove that an infection must be at least at the root of the rheumatoid disease problem."

[I find it most interesting — and consistent — that Dr. Pybus found 83% suffer a Herxheimer reaction, and subsequently show improvement or alleviation of this disease, and that Gus Prosch, Jr.[14], M.D. has shown a cure/remission rate of about 80% since 1982, using these oral medications combined with intraneurals and proper diet. This figure does not apply to those treated with traditional immuno-modulating drugs, as then our percentages of success drops to 50%: Ed.]

[It is stated and referenced in Roger Wyburn-Mason's[12] various works that The Herxheimer response only occurs when an organism more complex than a bacillus is being killed by an antibiotic and due to the Herxheimer, this fact "proves" that the infective agent must be of a complicated structure. Ed.]

"In South Africa, our research has been based on the effect of metronidazole on moving cells found in joint fluid. It has been shown that the macrophage-like cells found in the rheumatoid fluid, when challenged with metronidazole, first respond with an increased movement of a writhing character. These movements after 15 minutes largely subside to be replaced by the slower movement and eventually after 309 minutes they are mostly crenated and absorbed. Thus, the metronidazole would appear to kill the macrophage [*in vitro*: Ed.].

"Wyburn-Mason stressed that the *Amoeba chromatosa* was often confused with macrophages, and that they had the power of independent existence for a long time, which fact [of independent existence] some of us have corroborated." [Roger Wyburn-Mason and Vice Admiral protozoologist Stamm probably viewed clusters of cell-wall deficient bacteria: Ed.]

"Kwang Jeon[15] [University of Tennessee, U.S.A.] cultured these cells in joint fluid that were up to one week old and showed that they would develop into fibroblasts. However, the fluid that had been treated with metronidazole grew nothing.

"Davies[16] has noted these macrophages in penassy fluid left at room temperature were still fresh (active) for as long as 24 days.

"Wyburn-Mason[17] described the macrophage in great detail and gave it great prominence in his book on the reticuloendothelial system. He concluded it was not mesodermal in origin as is so often claimed and said, but not proved, to develop from the monocyte, but rather was it neuroectodermal in origin and was developed from the trophic nerve ending.

"Later, when working with Stamm[12], he was convinced that these were in all probability amoebae. Furthermore, they both claimed that they had cultured them, but attempts by all of us have failed to repeat this.

"However, these macrophages have been grown at the University of Tennessee by Kwang Jeon and this, I feel, is a great step forward."

"References to Dr. Paul K. Pybus Paper

1. Herxheimer, K. Krause: "Ubereine bei Syphilitische vorkommende Quecksilerberreaktion. *Deutsch. Med. Wschr.* 28:50, 1902.

2. Herxheimer, K. and Martin, H.: So-called Herxheimer reactions. *Arch. Derm. Syph.* 13:115, 1926.

3. Millian, G.: Syphilis: Reaction d' Herxheimer. *Biotropisme. Paris nd.*: 37:91, 1920.

4. Fleishman, K. and Kreibich, C.: Zum Wesen der Reaktion nach Jarish-Herxheimer. *Me. Klin.* 21:1157, 1925.

5. Mahoney, J.F., Arnold, R.C., and Harris, A.: Penicillin treatment of early syphilis. *Amer. J. Public Health* 33:1387, 1943.

6. Moore, J.E., Farmer, T.W. and Hoekenga, M.T.: Penicillin and the Jarisch-Herxheimer reaction in early, cardiovascular and nuerosyphilis. *rans. Ass. Amer. Phycns.* 61:176, 1948.

7. Joulia, P., Pautrizell, R., Texier, L. and Sebra, De.: La chute des eosinophiles sanguines apre une premiere injeciton de penicilline au cours de la syphilis primosecondaire: temoin du conflit antigene-anticorps. *ull. Soc. Franc. Derm. Syph.* 58:399, 1951.

8. Heyman, A., Sheldon, W.H. and Evans, L.D.:

Pathogenesis of the Jarisch-Herxheimer reaction. *rit. J. vener. Dis.* 28:50, 1952.

9. Jadassohn, J.: Beitrag zur Jarisch-Herxheimer Reaktion. *Z. Haut Geschlechtskr* 19:158, 1965.

10. Jarisch, A. Wien. *med Wschr.* 45:721, 1895.

11. Gudjonsson, Haraldur: The Jarisch-Herxheimer Reaction, Stockholm 1972 (A summary based on the following seven publications:

a. Skok, E. and Gudjonsson, H.: On the allergic origin of the jarisch-Herxheimer reaction. *Acta Dermatovfener* (Stockholm) 46:136, 1966.

b. Gudjonsson, H. and Skog, E.: The effect of prednisolone on the Jarisch-Herxheimer reaction. *Acta Dermatovener* (Stockholm) 48:15, 1968.

c. Gudjonsson, H. and Skog, E.: Fever after inoculation of rabbits with *Treponema pallidum.* Jarisch-Herxheimer reaction? *Proc. 18. Meeting Scand. Dermatol. Ass.*, Turku 1968.

d. Gudjonsson, H. and Skog, E.: Fever after inoculation of rabbits with *Treponema pallidum. Brit. J. vener. Dis.* 46:318, 1970.

e. Gudjonsson, H., Newman, B. and Turner, T.B.: Demonstration of a virus-like agent contaiminating amterial containing the Stockholm substrain of the Nichols pathogenic *Treponema pallidum. Brit. J. vener. Dis.* 46:435, 1970.

f. Gudjonsson, H. Newman, B. and Turner, T.B.: Screening out a virus-like agent from the testicular suspension of the Nichols pathogenic *Treponema pallidum. Brit. J. vener. Dis.* In press at time summary was written.

g. Gudjonsson, H.: Experiments to induce febrile Jarisch-Herxheimer reaction on syphilitic rabbits with penicillin and erythromycin. *Acta Dermatovener.* (Stockholm). In press at time summary was written.

12. Wyburn-Mason, Roger: *The Causation of Rheumatoid Disease and Many Human Cancers*, IJI Publishing Co., Ltd., Tokyo, Japan, 1978. [Summary available through The Rheumatoid Disease Foundation, Rt. 4, Box 137, Franklin, TN 37064, same title.]

13. See *Rheumatoid Diseases Cured at Last* (1985) or *The Art of Getting Well* (1988) both available through The Arthritis Trust of America, 7111 Sweetgum Drive SW, Fairview, TN 37062-9384.

14. Prosch, Gus J., Jr.: Personal communcation: Ed.

15. Jeon, Kwang: Research proposal and paper (based on arthritic knee effusion samples submitted by our referral physicians from their patients) submitted to The Rheumatoid Disease Foundation.

16. Pybus, Paul K. P, Davies, A.H.: Paper submitted to The Rheumatoid Disease Foundation (based on knee effusions submitted by our referral physicians.)

17. Wyburn-Mason, Roger: *The Reticulo-Endothellial System in Growth and Tumour Formation*, Henry Kimpton, London, England, 1958.

Other Considerations

The Arthritis Trust of America/The Rheumatoid Disease Foundation former referral physicians who have kept statistics since 1982 have achieved an 80% remission/cure rate from Rheumatoid Disease provided the patient has not already been treated with gold, penicillamine, methotrexate, cyclosporin, long-term cortico-steroids, or other damaging immuno-modulating drugs. If the patient has been treated by these immuno-modulating substances, then the recovery rate drops to 50%, which is still 30% more than those simply "improving" from traditional and established treatments[1,2].

Other physicians, with other modalities, such as herbal therapy or homeopathy have also been successful. It is believed that all successful treatments are related in assisting the restoration of the patient to an initial healthy state by a combination of known and unknown mechanisms.

As with Osteoarthritis, and aside from food allergies and nightshades (solanines), dietary considerations, including mineral and vitamin supplements and herbal usages, often emphasize characteristics of anti-oxidants, anti-inflammatories, synergisms with other substances, hormonal replacements or blockages, or faster re-growth of, or maintenance of connective tissue. As the immune system is presumed to have been compromised, strong strategies are often utilized in conjunction with diet and supplements to strengthen the immunological system. This includes the long-term replacement of organisms- of-opportunity found in the intestinal tract by friendly bacteria -- *Lactobacillus acidophilus* and *Bifido bacterium*[24].

Mineral and vitamin supplements include Selenium, Zinc, Manganese, Vitamin C, Proteolytic Enzymes, Flavonoids, D, L-Phenylalanine, Niacinamide, Tryptophan, Superoxide Dismutase, Panthothenic Acid, Sulfur (Cysteine), Methionine, Essential Fatty Acids[95], and Copper Aspirinate. [Seldon Nelson, M.D. developed resin-coated copper granules for sub-lingual usage that was reported successful[72]. Most of these are anti-inflammatory, anti-oxidant[22] or supplements for deficient nutritional substances. Rex E. Newnham[23], Ph.D., D.O., N.D. has reported excellent success in using Boron with both Osteoarthritis and Rheumatoid Disease Patients. Newnham[23] states that Boron plays a role in the retention of calcium and also positively stimulates hormonal factors. William Kaufman, Ph.D., M.D. has also reported similar success when using Niacinamide. Perhaps Boron and Niacinamide are somehow related in physiological processes[90, 91]. If so, there should be research literature avialable somewhere that demonstrates the relationship, thus giving us a better clue to causation of arthritides.

Dr. Thomas MacPherson Brown reported success in the use of Tetracycline, based on findings that mycoplasmas were isolated from a chimpanzee[74]. Many physicians do not like to use tetracycline as (1) they have not seen the reported good results, and (2) they feel that its use drastically increases Candidiasis[75].

Herbal medicines often recommended for arthritides are: *Curcuma longa, Zingiber Officinale, Tanacetum parthenium, Harpagophytum procumbens, Bupleuri falcatum, Glycyrrhiza glabra, Panax ginseng, Scutellaria baicalensis* and the proanthocyanidins, Blueberries, Cherries and Hawthorn Berries[22]. Many of these herbs simply dampen inflammation, but some may very well contribute to restoration of health in other ways.

Chapter V
A Case History

A 57 year old male (now 70), with stress from his job, marriage, and finances, developed progressively increasing symptoms of heated and swollen joints. He was filled with pain, lethargy and depression, and he often woke up nights finding his bed soaked with sweat. He was told by his family doctor that he had Rheumatoid Arthritis, that he would be crippled soon, and there was no hope, other than the temporary easing of pain and other symptoms by means of Non-Steroidal Anti-inflammatory drugs (NSAIDS); and later, as the disease progressed, use of cortisone, gold shots and then methotrexate. (Rheumatologists now seem to reverse this progression, starting first with damaging methotrexate.)

The idea of being crippled was perhaps the greater fear, and even deeper lethargy and depression set in.

Intuitively this patient knew that he had to relieve stress, and he took necessary steps to do so. There was also a sufficient spark of hope in this patient to continue to search for alternatives, and at last, after trying various home-folk remedies proferred by one friend or another, he found the treatment recommended by Roger Wyburn-Mason, M.D., Ph.D. and Jack M. Blount, M.D. Dr. Blount, himself a victim of crippling Rheumatoid Arthritis for many years, sympathetically taught this patient what do do, and which prescription medicines to take. Dr. Blount wrote prescriptions for metronidazole and allopurinol which the patient took, although his family doctor felt it would be safe but useless.

Within three days a severe Herxheimer effect occurred and, had the patient not been strongly warned of these consequences of taking his prescription medicines, he would have assumed that his Rheumatoid Arthritis was now flaring up in an extreme manner. More joints than before begin aching excrutiatingly, night sweats increased in severity, joints became more swollen and heated, and lethargy and depression had reached what he described as "the pits."

The Herxheimer effect tapered off during the next six weeks. It became clear to this patient that all the key characteristics of Rheumatoid Arthritis were gone: pyrexia (heat), edema (swelling), lethargy and depression, night sweats and an increasing number of painful joints.

There had been a great deal of damage to this patient during the period while Rheumatoid Disease was progressing, and so various joints still held pain. Dr. Paul Pybus, developer of Intra-Neural Injections visited America from Africa and between Dr. Pybus and Gus J. Prosch, Jr., M.D. (who learned and taught Pybus' technique), the patient began receiving intra-neurals every three to four months. The doctor would palpate -- touch with his finger -- key nerve ganglia near the surface of the skin. As these nerve ganglia led to joints with pain, whenever one was found with disturbed cellular nerve cell membranes, the doctors would mark the spots, and later inject them with a combination of Depot Medrol and a very dilute solution of Triamcinolone Hexacetonide, a pain killer and cellular membrane stabilizer. This combination of medicines, acting locally, not systemically, caused the pain in the joints to disappear immediately. Pybus's past evidence showed that such relief lasted anywhere from three months on up to five years. Over a period of two years, treatments taken three to six months apart, the patient observed that there were increasingly less painful nerve ganglia, and that the beneficial effects of the treatments lasted longer each time taken.

Also, every three to six months the patient had to repeat the prescription medicines, each time going through the Herxheimer effect, but not in the severe form first encountered, each Herxheimer lasting but a night, or at most, two nights.

After two years the patient at last heeded Dr. Gus Prosch's (and other physicians) advice to pay attention to diet and vitamin and mineral supplementation, including avoiding the wrong kind of fats and oils, and consuming the correct kind of essential fatty acids. He convinced himself to change his life-style based on the saliva litmus test designed by Carl Reiche, M.D., finding that his saliva invariably gave an extremely pale color indicating extreme acidic condition.

It was difficult for this patient to change his life style, as 59 years (by now) of education in faulty nutritional advice had led him to live on fast food hamburgers, candy bars and pop, canned goods, margarine and so on. As an experiment he studied the use of mega-dosages of vitamins and minerals, and grudgingly started eating fresh fruits, vegetables, whole grains and fresh-water fish. He also changed his cooking oils to that of Virgin Olive Oil, used butter rather than margarine, supplemented with a quality grade of Flaxseed Oil, and ate more nuts, such as walnuts, all according to Gus J. Prosch, M.D.'s advice.

While it took time to observe a difference, it eventually became clear that he no longer needed the intra-neural injections.

While the struggle to change diet continued, this same patient still suffered from extreme tiredness and claudication in the legs, a pronounced symptom of pain and cramping on lying down. He learned of EDTA Chelation Therapy, and also DMSO Intravenous (IV) Therapy, taking more than eighty-eight of the former and nine of the latter. It is clear from loss of specific symptoms and ease of exercise that this patient benefited greatly from these intravenous (IV) treatments.

The same patient tried oral Hydrogen Peroxide treatment, but could not tolerate the oral administration which produced in him extreme nausea.

He also learned that all Rheumatoid Disease victims suffer from Candidiasis by reason of having had a weakened immunological system, and so he sought advice and treatment against these organisms of opportunity, also learning to supplement with *Lactobaccilus acidolphilus* and *Bifido bacterium*, along with other vitamin, mineral and essential fatty acid supplements.

He found himself impotent, and after several trials and studies he twice injected bis-beta carboxyethyl germanium sesquioxide, Ge-132, which solved the impotency problem.

He successfully used the "pure water five-day diet" solving some difficult problems by permitting the body to detoxify in that manner, while also learning, by single food challenges, to which foods he was especially allergic.

Damage done to his body had resulted in extreme pain in the neck and shoulder which normally would have required spinal fusions. Fortunately, this same patient, being wise enough to search out additional alternatives, discovered reconstructive therapy (sclerotherapy or pro-liferative therapy) through William J. Faber, D.O. Dr. Faber referred him to James O. Carlson, D.O., who specializes in non-surgical sports medicine. Over the period of twelve months, one treatment per month, Dr. Carlson helped the patient restore his body's structure, pain-free. It should not have taken more than three to six months, but his basal metabolism was low. This he learned by the use of the Broda O. Barnes', M.D. armpit temperature measurement technique, and is now on thyroid replacement therapy additionally. As use of reconstructive therapy depends on the body's ability to repair itself, the basal metabolism must be functioning effectively for rapid success after treatment.

He completed a series of Rolfing massages, restoring his structural integrity, and which also reduced a great deal of pain in the left leg, leaving just a touch of tende-nonitis from instability aggravated by fast (swing; jitter-bug) dancing, which he still does, at age of 70, three or four times per week.

For a period he suffered from active gout, and took for several years Colbenamid™ (probenecid and colchicine) and allopurinol. How it finally resolved itself is unknown.

He tried Life Crystals (dna/rna/glucose) and Chondrianas (alleged precursors to mitochondria with ability to restore organs) as described by the Life Crystal Company, to no good effect, learning that there were no Chondrianas in the substances received, but rather danger-ous gram-negative bacteria.

He received live-cell therapy from Lester Winter, Ph.D. and found some temporary (1 year) improvement in a skin condition and in hypoglycemia (6 months).

From Susana Alcazar Leyva, M.D. he received injec-tions of a form of thiamine (cocarboxylase) and nicotinamide dinucleotide plus adenine. These self-administered shots, taken twice weekly (for 1 year), have greatly improved energy through, presumably, improvement of metabolic activity.

His left leg tendonitis problem had been intransigent for more than five years, and calcium spurs on his fingers are beginning to interfere with his ability to type. He's therefore exploring new means to solve these two problems. The use of ELF laboratory's Light Beam Generator seems to have solved his long-standing leg tendonitis problem, as well as long-standing, persistent pain in one finger.

He explored the usage of DHEA, as a replacement hormone, because of his age. He was delighted with the effects of this safe, replacement hormone, finding a great deal more energy.

He's is now exploring the applications and useage of herbology.

Despite bothersome Osteoarthritis and calcium spurs -- for which he's searching for answers -- the patient reports a renewed lease of life -- at least his quality of life -- and wants everyone to know what he's accomplished. He also wants folks to know that he's still got other problems stemming from prior damage done by the raging disease process, and also aging problems, accompanied with some long time mold and house-dust allergy problems. Nonetheless he follows the advice given in this book, to search out means for solving, not just alleviating, the symptoms[65]. He will probably investigate one thing or another, to sustain or improve quality of old age, until the day his whole system finally gives out, probably like the one-hoss shay, all at once.

One thing is clear: Rheumatoid Disease is a great crippler unless the individual is willing to search out and to use treatment modalities that are not otherwise accepted by the established medical doctrine; and further, that the patient be willing to take personal responsibility for his/her own recovery, not despairing because one doctor or one form of treatment is not successful, but rather going on to find the one suited to one's own unique condition.

The above case history is presented to demonstrate what can be done if you're determined to get well, and to improve the quality of your livingness.

Chapter VI
Gouty Arthritis
What Is Gouty Arthritis?

Gouty Arthritis is characterized by sharp painful joints, as if a needle were probing the internal structure of the joints. One can have attacks of fever, chills and, of course, the described excruciating needle-like pains. Gout victims will suffer for weeks at a time often with loss of mobility; and, as these attacks become more frequent, they will eventually be disabling. Kidney disease, heart disease, and many other complications can set in[5].

The nature of Gouty Arthritis is most easily understood and controlled, as it stems from a partially known set of causes. It is a defect in the ability to rid oneself of uric acid, thus causing uric acid crystals to lodge in the collagen tissue matrices throughout portions of the body, especially near and around the joints. It also causes kidney stones, high blood pressure and other health problems in some folks, but it rarely afflicts women or children. As Osteoporosis is predominately a woman's disease, gout is predominantely a man's disease, the ratio being about 19 men for 1 women. Ninety-five percent of gout victims, therefore, are men. The few women who have gout show signs and symptoms after menopause, so there must surely be a hormonal component to gout. Children are almost never affected[5].

Up until the 1960's gout was a terrible disease without much help from the medical profession. One had attacks of fever, chills and excruciating needle-like pains. The gout victim suffered for weeks at a time. Eventually the attacks of gout became more frequent and eventually disabling, with kidney disease, heart disease and many other complications setting in[5].

What Causes Gouty Arthritis?

Those who suffer from gout have a condition known as Hyperuricemia, which simply means too much uric acid in the blood serum. If you placed some of the patient's blood on a string and let it dry, there would form linked crystals of uric acid. These when deposited in the wrong places in the body create joint inflammation, kidney blockage and lumps called "tophi[5].."

Uric acid does not easily dissolve in water, and blood is composed mainly of water. One gram of salt will dissolve in about one-half teaspoon of water; one gram of sugar in about one-tenth teaspoon of water. To dissolve the same amount of uric acid takes at least two quarts of water!

We can easily produce uric acid, and our bodies are geared to conserving it, instead of excreting it freely through our kidneys with other waste products. The kidneys remove it from the blood, and then restore most of it back to the bloodstream so that it can go on to other organs for use. It may also be that many gout victims are more efficient in doing this filtering/restoring, but that is only speculation[5]..

The extra uric acid must lodge someplace, and that's where the pain comes in, when the body decides to deposit the small uric acid crystals in a collagen matrix, especially near a moving joint.

How Can Gouty Arthritis Be Prevented And/Or

Treated?

Very little is known about what starts and stops gout attacks. Emotional upset or stress can surely bring on an attack. Without question, diet can control attacks, causing it to be greater or lesser depending upon what is eaten. Perhaps weather changes or drugs may precipitate an attack. There are no general rules that apply to everyone[5].

Besides the diet — and probably related to the diet — is the fact of tissue acidity/alkalinity balances.

It is also important that sufficient thyroid be produced or available to the metabolism.

Not enough is known about the metabolic defects that bring about gout and so, other than inheriting a healthy metabolism, and/or maintaining other healthy conditions, such as diet and relief of stress, appropriate physical exercise and so on, few recommendations can be given for preventing the condition known as Gouty Arthritis. At least one person -- and probably more than one -- has restored his bodily functions to a healthy condition and found that his gout had disappeared[55].

If you do find yourself with Gouty Arthritis, there is a well-known and accepted diet and medications that can be used to control the affliction. However, be careful with excessive weight-loss diet, as according to Warren Levin, M.D., "One of the well-recognized triggers for attacks of gout is a weight-reduction program emphasizing low carbohydrate. This results in the patient going into ketosis as the body burns fatty-acid residues for energy. [Ketosis is a condition of too many ketones in the body, any compound containing the carbonyl group, CO.]These are ordinarily harmless `clinkers' from the body's energy furnaces, although in excess they cause ketoacidosis as, for instance, severe diabetes where the body is unable to burn carbohydrates as well. The normal mechanism of excretion of ketone bodies is through the kidney and, hence, Dr.

Robert Atkins' use of KetoStix™ to prove the compliance of his patients on the rigorous carbohydrate restriction. This same excretory pathway, however, is utilized by the body in excreting uric acid. When there is a high level ketoacid, it's like competition for a revolving door, everything slows down. The result is sometimes a dramatic increase in serum levels of uric acid, which can precipitate either kidney stones or a gouty attack[97]."

Diet [5]

According to John Baron, D.O.[5], the Gouty Arthritic should avoid foods with a high purine content. These include all organ meats (liver, kidneys, sweetbreads, etc.), anchovies, gravies, meat extracts, salmon (and Lox, etc.), and sardines. Organ meats are often used in preparing sausages, luncheon meats and similar products. Avoid all alcoholic beverages[5].

Be careful with those of a fairly high purine content, such as asparagus, beans, peas, lentils, bran, celery, fish (freshwater and saltwater), meats (except organs mentioned above), mushrooms, oatmeal, poultry, radishes, seafood (crabs, oysters, lobsters), spinach, and wheatgerm[5]..

You can enjoy these: All vegetables except those mentioned above, breads and cereals (except whole grain), eggs, fats and oils, fish roe including caviar, gelatin, milk and milk products, nuts, sugars, syrups, and sweets[5]..

While the diet most often recommended for gout restricts the substances from which uric acid is formed; i.e. purines, some believe that the basic problem lies with inefficient breakdown of proteins in the body. However, if one chooses the low-purine diet, panthothenic acid (B_5) is necessary for conversion of uric acid into urea and ammonia., according to John D. Kirschmann and Lavon J. Dunne[108]. They say that "Stress rapidly depletes pantothenic acid as well as other B vitamins," and that "A lack of vitamin E allows excessive formation of uric acid. A diet of incomplete proteins or one too high or too low in isolated amino acids can also produce too much uric acid. They also recommend Vitamin A, Vitamin B complex, Vitamin B_1, Vitamin C (up to 5000 mg) , Calcium, Magnesium, Phosphorus, Potassium, Complete Protein, and *Lactobacillus acidophilus*. While iron is also recommended, this writer believes that sufficient evidence exists to support the thesis that we already receive too much iron.

James F. Balch, M.D. and Phyllis A. Balch, C.N.C.[109] in addition to vitamins and minerals recommends the use of Kelp which, they say, "Contains complete protein and vital minerals to reduce serum uric acid," and also bis beta-carboxyethyl germanium sesquioxide (Ge-132) which is "good for pain and swelling." (Other forms of germanium, such as germanium oxide, of course, are to be avoided as toxic; whereas this form acts as an electronic sink at the mitochodrial level in the cells, and is not absorbed by human tissue[57].) Superoxide dismutase is recommended as an antioxidant and potent free radical destroyer, and also zinc as important in protein metabolism and tissue repair[109].

Drugs and Herbs

Two medicines used to control gout are allopurinol and colchicine. Allopurinol keeps the body from lodging the crystals in collagen tissue and colchicine helps the body to dissolve the crystals already formed[5].

As various herbal preparations also contain the same or similar ingredients, often herbal remedies have been, and can be, used, toward the same ends.

Chapter VII

Physical Therapy

Physical therapy and/or heat is often given a major role in the treatment or management of arthritis. Certainly it is important to exercise sufficiently to keep the joints working, and for basic health, but a word of caution: In the case of Gouty Arthritis, such physical activity is not only extremely painful, but may also help to rapidly erode joint bearing surfaces by the action of uric acid crystals gouging into the surfaces.

In the case of Osteoarthritis, it may be most beneficial to limit exercise, and through rest to permit inflamed joints to dampen down.

If Rheumatoid Arthritis is caused by a genetic susceptibility to the protein products or toxins of an unknown organism[29], then extended exercise and heat will cause that organism to be spread further and faster, probably resulting in what is known as "galloping arthritis[51]." *The Rheumatoid Disease Foundation* takes the position that one should first halt the progress of the disease, and then conduct more strenuous exercises.

According to Robert Bingham, M.D. the arthritic should not strain unstable joints such as fingers, elbows, knees or ankles. "If your hands are affected, avoid old, stressful ways of opening jars, wringing out laundry, etc. Instead use a jar opener and other helpful tools to reduce stress on joints. Use tools with large handles. Use the palm of your hands for lifting and pushing. Push instead of pulling. Dishwashing should be done with fingers kept straight as much as possible. If a dishwasher is available use it in preference to washing by hand[20]."

Dr. Bingham also answers the question as to whether or not sexual activity will make arthritis worse. He says, "At the Moss Rehabilitation Hospital in Philadelphia, research on this very question reveals the following results as reported by Dr. George Ehrlich of Temple University Medical School[20].

"The sex act releases a hormone that acts like cortisone, probably from stimulation of the adrenal glands.

This may relieve pain and stiffness in specific parts of the body, such as the muscles and joints, and the beneficial effects may last up to 6 hours. The brain also releases hormones (endomorphins) into the blood stream that are also pain-relieving substances.

"*Any* form of exercise -- as sexual activity certainly is -- improves the circulation of the entire body. It speeds up breathing, the pulse rate, and the rate of circulating blood; it increases oxygen to the muscles and joints; and it improves joint motion and flexibility. All these body functions benefit the arthritis patient.

"However, sexual activity may be uncomfortable to some patients, who will seek body positions and sexual activities that are stimulating but not too uncomfortable.

"There is no medical evidence of sexual activity causing injury or making arthritis worse. On the contrary, it is on the recommended list of functions for arthritis patients[20]."

Text References
(Excluding those given within chapters)

1. Anthony di Fabio, *Rheumatoid Diseases Cured at Last*, The Arthritis Trust of America, 7111 Sweetgum Drive SW, Suite A, Fairview, TN 37062-9384, 1985; also see Kindle or Nook.

2. Anthony di Fabio, *The Art of Getting Well*, The Arthritis Trust of America, 7111 Sweetgum Drive SW, Fairview, TN 37062-9384, 1988; also see Kindle or Nook.

3. Anthony di Fabio, *Treatment and Prevention of Osteoarthritis*, Part I, The Arthritis Trust of America, 7111 Sweetgum Drive SW, Suite A, Fairview, TN 37062-9384, 1989. Also in *Townsend Letter for Doctors*, January 1990, #78; also Anthony di Fabio, *Arthritis*, The Arthritis Trust of America, 7111 Sweetgum Drive SW, Suite A, Fairview, TN 37062-9384.

4. Anthony di Fabio, *Treatment and Prevention of*

116

Osteoarthritis, Part II, The Arthritis Trust of America, 7111 Sweetgum Drive SW, Suite A, Fairview, TN 37062-9384, 1989. Also in *Townsend Letter for Doctors*, February/March 1990, #79/80; also Anthony di Fabio, *Arthritis*, The Arthritis Trust of America, 7111 Sweetgum Drive SW, Suite A, Fairview, TN 37062-9384.

5. Anthony di Fabio, *Gouty Arthritis*, The Arthritis Trust of America, 7111 Sweetgum Drive SW, Suite A, Fairview, TN 37062-9384, 1989.

6. Anthony di Fabio, *The Master Regulator*, The Arthritis Trust of America, 7111 Sweetgum Drive SW, Suite A, Fairview, TN 37062-9384, 1989.

7. Paul Pybus, *Intraneural Injections for Rheumatoid Arthritis and Osteoarthritis and The Control of Pain in Arthritis of the Knee*, The Arthritis Trust of America, 7111 Sweetgum Drive SW, Suite A, Fairview, TN 37062-9384, 1989.

8. William J. Faber, D.O. and Morton Walker, D.P.M., *Pain, Pain Go Away*, Milwaukee Pain Clinic & Metabolic Research Center, 6529 W. Fond du Lac Ave., Milwaukee, WI 53218, 1990.

9. William J. Faber, D.O. and Morton Walker, D.P.M., *Instant Pain Relief*, Milwaukee Pain Clinic & Metabolic Research Center, 6529 W. Fond du Lac Ave., Milwaukee, WI 53218, 1990.

10. James A. Carlson, D.O., Knoxville, TN.

11. John H. Klippel, M.D., John L. Decker, M.D. Ed., *Clinics in Rheumatic Diseases*, Vol. 9/No. 3, W.B. Saunders Company Ltd., December 1983.

12. L. Ron Hubbard, *Dianetics: The Modern Science of Mental Health*, Bridge Publications, Inc., 4751 Fountain Avenue, Los Angeles, CA 90029.

13. Perry A. Chapdelaine, Sr., "Herxheimer Reaction," *Townsend Letter for Doctors*, May 1991, #94.

14. Anthony di Fabio, *A Treatment for Scleroderma*

& *Lupus Erythematosus*, The Arthritis Trust of America, 7111 Sweetgum Drive SW, Fairview, TN 37062-9384, 1989. Also in *Townsend Letter for Doctors*, Dec. 1989, #77.

15. Anthony di Fabio, *The Surprising Psoriasis Treatment*, The Arthritis Trust of America, 7111 Sweetgum Drive SW, Suite A, Fairview, TN 37062-9384, 1989. Also in *Townsend Letter for Doctors*, June 1990, #83.

16. Peter Dosch, M.D. *Manual of Neural Therapy according to Huneke*, Eleventh Edition, Haug Publishers., 1984.

17. Pizzorno & Murray, *Textbook of Natural Medicine*, Osteoarthritis VI: Osteoa-1 , 1991.

18. Pizzorno & Murray, *Textbook of Natural Medicine*, Rheumatoid Arthritis VI: RA-4, 1991.

19. Pizzorno & Murray, *Textbook of Natural Medicine*, Rheumatoid Arthritis VI: RA-5, 1991. 1985.

21. Anthony di Fabio, *Essential Fatty Acids are Essential,* The Arthritis Trust of America, 7111 Sweetgum Drive SW, Suite A, Fairview, TN 37062-9384, 1989. Also see Pizzorno & Murry, RA-4, 1991.

22. Pizzorno & Murray, *Rheumatoid Arthritis* VI: RA-4-5 1991.

23. Rex E. Newnham, Ph.D., D.O., N.D., *Away With Arthritis,* Cracoe House Cottage, Cracoe, Skipton, North Yorkshire BD23 6LB England.

24. Anthony di Fabio, *Friendly Bacteria -- Lactobacillus acidophilus & Bifido bacterium*, The Arthritis Trust of America, 7111 Sweetgum Drive SW, Suite A, Fairview, TN 37062-9384.

25. Richard Edelson, Peter Heald, Maritza Perez, Alain Rook, "Photopheresis Update," *Progress in Dermatology*, Vol. 25, No. 3, Sept. 1991.

26. Personal communication from William Campbell Douglass, M.D.

27. Personal visit in the U.S. with Tonis Pai, M.D.

28. Personal visit with Gus Prosch, Jr., M.D., Birmingham, AL.

29. Roger Wyburn-Mason, M.D., Ph.D., *The Causation of Rheumatoid Disease and Many Human Cancers*, The Arthritis Trust of America, 7111 Sweetgum Drive SW, Suite A, Fairview, TN 37062-9384, 1985.

30. Anthony di Fabio, *Bee Pollen: The Perfect Food*, The Arthritis Trust of America, 7111 Sweetgum Drive SW, Suite A, Fairview, TN 37062-9384.

31. Anthony di Fabio, *Hydrogen Peroxide Therapy*, The Arthritis Trust of America, 7111 Sweetgum Drive SW, Suite A, Fairview, TN 37062-9384.

32. Ed McCabe, *Oxygen Therapies*, Energy Publications, 99-RD1, Morrisville, NY 13408, 1988.

33. Broda O. Barnes, M.D., Lawrence Galton, *Hypothyroidism: The Unsuspected Illness*, Harper & Row, New York, 1976.

34. Walter O. Grotz, *Grotz: Hydrogen: Bibliography*, ECHO, 300 South 4th Street, Delano, MN 55328.

35. Personal Communication from Helmut Christ, M.D., Germany and William Campell Douglass, III, M.D., Georgia.

36. John E. Croft, L.R.C.S., F.R.S.H., *Natural Relief From Arthritis*, Nutri-Books, Box 5793, Denver Colorado 80217, 1979.

37. Kurt Donsbach, D.C., Ph.D. *Hydrogen Peroxide*.

38. Theron G. Randolph, M.D., Ralph W. Moss, Ph.D., *An Alternative Approach to Allergies*, Bantam Books, 1982.

39. Charles Marchand, *The Therapeutical Applications of Hydrozone and Glycozone*, Echo, Inc. PO Box 126 Delano, MN 55328, republished from the 1904 18th edition 1989.

40. Corazon Illarina, M.D., unpublished manuscript,

The Holistic Book Project, Inc. 436 N. Oakhurst Drive, Apt. A, Beverly Hills, CA 90210, 1992.

41. C. Orian Truss, M.D., *The Missing Diagnosis*, C. Orian Truss, 2614 Highland Avenue, Birmingham, AL 35205, 1982.

42. William G. Crook, M.D., *The Yeast Connection*, Third Edition, Professional Books, PO Box 3494, Jackson, TN 38301, 1986.

43. William G. Crook, M.D., Laura Stevens, *Solving the Puzzle of Your Hard-To-Raise Child*, Professional Books, PO Box 846, Jackson, TN 38302, 1987.

44. Morton Walker, D.P.M. "The Carnivora Cure for Cancer, AIDS & Other Pathologies," *Townsend Letter for Doctors*, p. 412, June 1991; and "The Carnivora Cure for Cancer, AIDS & Other Pathologies -- Part II", *Townsend Letter for Doctors*, 911 Tyler Street, Port Townsend, WA 98368-6541, p. 329, May 1992.

45. Royden Brown, "Bee Pollen Cure for COPD," *Townsend Letter for Doctors*, 911 Tyler Street, Port Townsend, WA 98368-6541, p. 500, June 1992.

46. Personal communication with Royden Brown, Renaissance Laboratories, 3627 E. Indian School Road, Suite 209, Phoenix, AZS 85018.

47. Theron G. Randolph, M.D. & Ralph W. Moss, Ph.D., *An Alternative Approach to Allergies*, Bantam Book, July 1982.

48. *The Purification Rundown*, Bridge Publications, Inc., 1414 North Catalina Street, Los Angeles, CA 90027.

49. David W. Schnare, Max Ben, Megan G. Shields, "Body Burden Reductions of PCBs, PBBs and Chlorinated Pesticides in Human Subjects," *Ambio* Vol. 13, NO. 5-6, p. 378, 1984.

50. Ziga Tretjack, Megan Shields, Shelley L. Beckmann, "PCB Reduction and Clinical Improvement by Detoxification: An Unexploited Approach?" *Human &*

Experimental Toxicology **9**, 235-244, 1990.

51. Human Detoxification: New Hope for Firefighters, *California Fire Fighter*, Federated Fire Fighters of California, No. 4, 1984.

52. Personal experience, Perry A. Chapdelaine, Sr.

53. Buryl Payne, Ph.D., *The Body Magnetic*, 4264 Topsail Ct., Soquel, CA 95073, from "Book Notices," *Townsend Letter for Doctors,* April 1993, p. 270.

54. Hal A. Huggins, D.D.S., *It's All In Your Head*, Life Sciences Press, 4th Edition, 1990.

55. Royden Brown, *How to Live The Millenium*, Pains Corporation, Phoenix, AZ 85018.

56. "Goodbye Candida," Nutri-Dyn, Nu Biologics, 2470 Wisconsin Street, Downers Grove, IL 60515-4019.

57. Anthony di Fabio, *Germanium*, The Arthritis Trust of America, 7111 Sweetgum Drive SW, Suite A, Fairview, TN 37062-9384.

58. Sandra Goodman, Ph.D., *Germanium, The Health and Life Enhancer*, Thorsons Publishers Limited, Wellingborough, Northamptonshire, NN8 2RQ England.

59. Betty Kamen, Ph.D. *Germanium: A New Approach to Immunity*, Nutrition Encounter, Inc., Box 689, Larkspur, CA 94939.

60. Penny C. Royal, *Herbally Yours*, Sound Nutrition, 2560 North 560 East, Provo, UT 84604, 1987.

61. Yoshide Hagiwara, M.D. *Green Barley Essence*, Keats Publishing Co, 27 Pine St. (Box 876), New Canaan, CT 06840, 1985.

62. Maureen Salaman, *Nutrition: The Cancer Answer*, Stratford Publishing, 1259 El Camino Real, Suite 1500, Menlo Park, CA 94025, 1983.

63. Nathan Pritikin, *The Pritikin Promise*, Pocket Books, Simon & Schuster, Inc., 1985.

64. Linus Pauling, *How To Live Longer and Feel Better*, Avon Books, 105 Madison Ave., New York, NY

10016, 1986.

65. The Rheumatoid Disease Foundation files.

66. Harvey Bigelsen, M.D., *The Townsend Letter for Doctors*, #51, p. 294, Oct. 1987.

67. Ralph Wilson, Abstracter, of Callinan, P. "The Mechanism of Action of Homeopathic Remedies -- Towards a Definitive Mode of Action," *J. of Complementry Medicine*, July 1985.

68. Dr. Erik Enby, *Hidden Killers*, Peter Gosch, Michael Sheehan, Sheehan Communications, 1990.

69. Luc De Schepper, M.D., Ph.D., C.A., Peak Immunity, 2901 Wilshire Boulevard, Suite 435, Santa Monica, CA 90403, 1989.

70. "British Medical Journal Acknowledges the Value of Homeopathy," *The Townsend Letter for Doctors*, #96, July 1991.

71. Dennis W. Remington, M.D., Barbara W. Higa, R.D., *Back to Health*, Vitality House International, Inc., 3707 North Canyon Road #8-C, Provo, UT 84604.

72. Seldon Nelson, M.D., "The Use of Ionic Copper in the Treatment of Arthritis," *The Journal of the Academy of Rheumatoid Diseases*, Volume I, No. 3, Robert Bingham, M.D., 7750 Katella Ave., Suite 203, Stanton, CA 90680, 1987.

73. Raymond F. Peat, Ph.D., "Hormone Balancing: Natural Treatment," *The Journal of the Rheumatoid Disease Medical Association*, Volume 1, Number 1, Robert Bingham, M.D., 7750 Katella Ave., Suite 203, Stanton, CA 90680, 1986.

74. Robert Bingham, M.D., "The Arthritis Program of the Desert Arthritis Medical Clinic," *The Journal of the Rheumatoid Disease Medical Association*, Volume 2, Number 1, Robert Bingham, M.D., 7750 Katella Ave., Suite 203, Stanton, CA 90680, 1990.

75. Based on reports over 10 years to The Rheumatoid

122

Disease Foundation.

76. Reproductions of *The Microzymas and The Blood* (1908) translated by Montague Leverson, M.D. (1911) available through John & Frieda Mattingly, PO Box 7178, Loveland, CA 80537.

77. Personal Visitation to Lida Mattman, Ph.D. and author of definitive work, *Cell Wall Deficient Organisms,* Chemical Rubber Company Press (Out of print); and also *Cell Wall Deficient Forms Stealth Pathogens,* 2nd Edition, Chemical Rubber Company Press, Boca Raton, FL 1993.

78. Gerald J. Domingue, Jorgen U. Schlegel, Hannah B. Woody, "Naked Bacteria in Human Blood," *Microbia,* Tome 2, No. 2, 1976.

79. Arabinda Das, M.D. "A Doctor's Case: What Happens When a Physician Becomes a Rheumatoid Arthritis Patient?" *The Townsend Letter for Doctors,* July 1992.

80. Jeffrey S. Bland, Ph.D. "Managing Endo- and Exotoxicity," *Townsend Letter for Doctors,* July 1992.

81. American Apitherapy Society, Inc., Letters to the Editors, *The Townsend Letter for Doctors,* p. 610, July 1992.

82. Zane R. Gard, M.D. and Erma J. Brown, BSN, Ph.N. "Literature Review & Comparison Studies of the Sauna and Illness -- Part II," *The Townsend Letter for Doctors,* July 1992.

83. Virginia Livingston-Wheeler, Edmond G. Addeo, *The Conquest of Cancer,* Franklin Watts, 1984.

84. John W. Mattingly, *Microscopy, Bacteriology and Gaston Naessens' Biological Theory,* 2408 Frances Drive, Loveland, CO 80537, Jan. 1986.

85. Raul Vergini, M.D., "Magnesium Chloride in Acute and Chronic Diseases," *The Townsend Letter for Doctors,* No v. 1992, p. 992.

86. Ida P. Rolf, Ph.D., *Rolfing The Integration of Human Structures*, Harper & Row Publishers, 1977.

87. Rolf Institute, PO Box 1868, Boulder, CO 80306.

88. Personal communication with Thomas Gervais.

89. William Kaufman, Ph.D., M.D.,"The Use of Vitamin Therapy to Reverse Certain Concomitants of Aging," *Journal of the American Geriatrics Society*, Vol. III, No. 11, Nov. 1955, p. 927-936.

90. William Kaufman, Ph.D., M.D. "Niacinamide: A Most Neglected Vitamin," *Journal of the International Academy of Preventive Medicine*, Vol. VIII, No. 1, Winter, 1983.

91. William Kaufman, Ph.D., M.D. *The Common Form of Joint Dysfunction*, E.L. Hildreth & Co., 1949.

92. Personal communication with Rolfer Les Kertay, M.A.

93. Lester Winters, M.D., *Cellular Therapy*, Cellular Therapy Physician Associates of Tijuana, Tijuana, Baja California, Mexico, address mail to 2182 March Place, San diego, CA 92110. Also personal communication with Lester Winters, M.D.

94. Gerhard Shettler, Prof. Dr. med. "Intra-articular Cellular Therapy and Adjunctive Treatment," University of Cologne, Bundesreupublik Deutchland.

95. Personal communication with Gus J. Prosch, Jr., M.D.

96. Julian Whitaker, M.D. *Health & Healing*, Vol. 2, No.6., June 1992.

97. Warren Levin, M.D. Personal Communication.

98. Anthony di Fabio, *Chelation Therapy*, The Arthritis Trust of America, 7111 Sweetgum Drive SW, Suite A, Fairview, TN 37062-9384.

99. Anthony di Fabio, *The Herxheimer Effect*, The Arthritis Trust of America, 7111 Sweetgum Drive SW, Suite A, Fairview, TN 37062-9384.

124

100. Personal visit to William J. Saccoman, M.D. clinic and to Lester J. Winter, M.D.

101. Webster's New Universal Unabridged Dictionary.

102. Robert R. Barefoot, Carl J. Reich, M.D., *The Calcium Factor*, Bokar Consultants, Inc., PO Box 21270, Wickenburg, AZ 85358, 1992.; also personal letters from Carl J. Reich, M.D. to The Rheumatoid Disease Foundation.

103. *The Key to the Power of Vitamin C*, Inter-Cal Corporation, 421 Miller Valley Road, Prescott, AZ 86301.

104. William H. Philpott, M.D., Dean R. Bonlie, D.D.S., *The Magnetics of Stress Evoked Cellular Injury and Disease and Anti-stress Controlled Health Maintenance and Healing*, Philpott Medical Services, 17171 S.E. 29th Street, Choctaw, OK 73020, Oct. 1992.

105 . Personal correspondence from Carl J. Reich, M.D. to Perry A. Chapdelaine, Sr., December 27, 1992.

106. Gerald J. Domingue, Jorgen U. Schlegel, Hannah B. Woody, "Naked Bacteria in Human Blood," *Microbia,* Tome 2, No. 2, Annee 1976.

107. Dr. Julian Whitaker, "DHEA References," *Health & Healing*," June 1992; also see "DHEA: The Closest We Can Get, Today, To A Foundation of Youth," Op.Cit., Vol.2, No. 6, June 1992; William Regelson, Roger Loria, Mohammed Kalimi, "Hormonal Intervention: `Buffer Hormones' or `State Dependency,' Neuroimmunomodulation: Intervention in Aging and Cancer," *Annales N.Y. Acad. Sci.,* Vol. 521, 1988; George Weber, Ed., "Advances in Enzyme Regulation," *Proceedings of the Twenty-Sixth Symposium on Regulation of Enzyme Activity and Synthesis in Normal and Neoplastic Tissues held at Indiana University School of Medicine, Indianapolis, Indiana,* Volume 26, Pergamon Press, September 29, 30, 1986; Jonathan V. wright, M.D., *Physi-*

ologic and `Supraphysiologic' Suppression of Allergy by Dehydroepiandrosterone, February 26, 1990.

108. John D. Kirschmann, Lavon J. Dunne, *Nutrition Almanac*, 2nd Edition, McGraw-Hill Book Company, 1984, p. 158..

109. James F. Balch, M.D., Phyllis A. Balch, C.N.C., *Prescription for Nutritional Healing*, Avery Publishing Group, Inc., Garden City Park, New York, 1990, p. 191.

110. Rex E. Newnham Ph.D., D.O., N.D., Personal correspondence to Perry A. Chapdelaine, Sr., February 25, 1993, and also see *Osteo Trace* label, Mumme Enterprises, 1321 Meridian Avenue, South Pasadena, CA 91030.

111. Robert W. Bradford, D.Sc., Henry W. Allen, Michael L. Culbert, D.Sc., *The Biochemical Basis of Live Cell Therapy,*" The Robert Bradford Foundation, 1180 Walnut avenue, Chula Vista, California, 92011-2622, May 1986.

112. William H. Philpott, M.D., *Magnetic Research Protocols*, Philpott Medical Services, 17171 S.E. 29th Street, Choctaw, OK 73020.

113. Courtland Reeves, Fax Letter received from ELF Laboratories, 1314 Burch Drive, Evansville, IN 47711, January 1994.

114. R.O. Becker, "The BAsic Biological Data Transmission and Control System Influenced by Electrical Forces," *Ann. N.Y. Acad. Sci.* Vol. 238, pp. 236, 1974.

115. W.R. Adey, "Tissue Interactions with Non-Ionizing Electromagnetic Fields," *Physiol. Rev.*, Vol. 61, pp 435, 1981.

116. Ilanka Harezi, "The Danger of the Magnet Buzz," *Explore*, Vol. 4, No. 3 and 4, 1993, p. 128. Also write to ELF Laboratories, 1314 Burch Drive, Evansville, IN 47711 for further information, or copy of the article itself.

Books and Other Reading Materials

1. Anthony di Fabio, *Rheumatoid Diseases Cured at*

126

Last, The Arthritis Trust of America, 7111 Sweetgum Drive SW, Suite A, Fairview, TN 37062-9384, 1985.

2. Anthony di Fabio, *The Art of Getting Well*, The Arthritis Trust of America, 7111 Sweetgum Drive SW, Suite A, Fairview, TN 37062-9384, 1988.

3. Anthony di Fabio, *Treatment and Prevention of Osteoarthritis*, Part I, The Arthritis Trust of America, 7111 Sweetgum Drive SW, Suite A, Fairview, TN 37062-9384, 1989. Also in *Townsend Letter for Doctors*, January 1990, #78.

4. Anthony di Fabio, *Treatment and Prevention of Osteoarthritis*, Part II, The Arthritis Trust of America, 7111 Sweetgum Drive SW, Suite A, Fairview, TN 37062-9384, 1989. Also in *Townsend Letter for Doctors*, February/March 1990, #79/80.

5. Anthony di Fabio, *Gouty Arthritis*, The Arthritis Trust of America, 7111 Sweetgum Drive SW, Suite A, Fairview, TN 37062-9384, 1989.

6. Anthony di Fabio, *The Master Regulator*, The Arthritis Trust of America, 7111 Sweetgum Drive SW, Suite A, Fairview, TN 37062-9384, 1989.

7. Paul Pybus, *Intraneural Injections for Rheumatoid Arthritis and Osteoarthritis and The Control of Pain in Arthritis of the Knee*, The Arthritis Trust of America, 7111 Sweetgum Drive SW, Suite A, Fairview, TN 37062-9384, 1989.

8. William J. Faber, D.O. and Morton Walker, D.P.M., *Pain, Pain Go Away*, Milwaukee Pain Clinic & Metabolic Research Center, 6529 W. Fond du Lac Ave., Milwaukee, WI 53218, 1990.

9. William J. Faber, D.O. and Morton Walker, D.P.M., *Instant Pain Relief*, Milwaukee Pain Clinic & Metabolic Research Center, 6529 W. Fond du Lac Ave., Milwaukee, WI 53218, 1990.

10. John H. Klippel, M.D., John L. Decker, M.D. Ed.,

Clinics in Rheumatic Diseases, Vol. 9/No. 3, W.B. Saunders Company Ltd., December 1983.

11. Anthony di Fabio, *Essential Fatty Acids are Essential,* The Arthritis Trust of America, 7111 Sweetgum Drive SW, Suite A, Fairview, TN 37062-9384, 1989.

12. Perry A. Chapdelaine, Sr., "Herxheimer Reaction," *Townsend Letter for Doctors*, May 1991, #94.

13. Anthony di Fabio, *A Treatment for Scleroderma & Lupus Erythematosus,* The Arthritis Trust of America, 7111 Sweetgum Drive SW, Suite A, Fairview, TN 37062-9384, 1989. Also in *Townsend Letter for Doctors*, Dec. 1989, #77.

14. Anthony di Fabio, *The Surprising Psoriasis Treatment,* The Arthritis Trust of America, 7111 Sweetgum Drive SW, Suite A, Fairview, TN 37062-9384, 1989. Also in *Townsend Letter for Doctors*, June 1990, #83.

15. Peter Dosch, M.D. *Manual of Neural Therapy According to Huneke*, Eleventh Edition, Haug Publishers., 1984.

16. Robert Bingham, M.D. *Fight Back Against Arthritis*, The Arthritis Trust of America, 7111 Sweetgum Drive SW, Suite A, Fairview, TN 37062-9384, 1985.

17. Jack M. Blount, M.D. Archimedes Concon, M.D., James Rowland, D.O., William Renforth, M.D., Paul Williamson, M.D., Roger Wyburn-Mason, M.D. *Historical Documents In Search of the Cure for Rheumatoid Disease*, The Arthritis Trust of America, 7111 Sweetgum Drive SW, Suite A, Fairview, TN 37062-9384, 1985.

18. Joan Wyburn-Mason, *Dedication, Love and Humour*, The Arthritis Trust of America, 7111 Sweetgum Drive SW, Suite A, Fairview, TN 37062-9384, 1985.

18. Roger Wyburn-Mason, M.D., Ph.D., *The Causation of Rheumatoid Disease and Many Human Cancers*, The Arthritis Trust of America, 7111 Sweetgum Drive SW, Suite A, Fairview, TN 37062-9384,1985.

128

19. Broda O. Barnes, M.D. and Lawrence Galton, *Hypothyroidism: The Unsuspected Illness* Harper & Row, New York 1976.

20. Rex E. Newnham, Ph.D., D.O., N.D., *Away With Arthritis,* Cracoe House Cottage, Cracoe, Skipton, North Yorkshire BD23 6LB England.

21. Pizzorno & Murray, *Textbook of Natural Medicine*, Osteoarthritis VI, 1991.

22. Pizzorno & Murray, *Textbook of Natural Medicine*, Rheumatoid Arthritis VI, 1991.

23. Anthony di Fabio, *Friendly Bacteria -- Lactobacillus acidophilus & Bifido bacterium*, The Arthritis Trust of America, 7111 Sweetgum Drive SW, Suite A, Fairview, TN 37062-9384.

24. Dr. Erik Enby, *Hidden Killers*, Peter Gosch, Michael Sheehan, Sheehan Communications, 1990.

25. Anthony di Fabio, *Hydrogen Peroxide Therapy*, The Arthritis Trust of America, 7111 Sweetgum Drive SW, Suite A, Fairview, TN 37062-9384.

26. Ed McCabe, *Oxygen Therapies*, Energy Publications, 99-RD1, Morrisville, NY 13408, 1988.

27. Dr. Lester Winters, *Cellular Therapy*, 2182 March Place, San Diego, CA 92110.

28. John E. Croft, L.R.C.S., F.R.S.H., *Natural Relief From Arthritis*, Nutri-Books, Box 5793, Denver Colorado 80217, 1979.

29. Kurt Donsbach, D.C., Ph.D. *Hydrogen Peroxide*,

30. Theron G. Randolph, M.D., Ralph W. Moss, Ph.D., *An Alternative Approach to Allergies*, Bantam Books, 1982.

31. Charles Marchand, *The Therapeutical Applications of Hydrozone and Glycozone*, Echo, Inc. PO Box 126 Delano, MN 55328, republished from the 1904 18th edition 1989.

32. C. Orian Truss, M.D., *The Missing Diagnosis*, C.

Orian Truss, 2614 Highland Avenue, Birmingham, AL 35205, 1982.

33. William G. Crook, M.D., *The Yeast Connection*, Third Edition, Professional Books, PO Box 3494, Jackson, TN 38301, 1986.

34. William G. Crook, M.D., Laura Stevens, *Solving the Puzzle of Your Hard-To-Raise Child*, Professional Books, PO Box 846, Jackson, TN 38302, 1987.

35. *Townsend Letter for Doctors*, 911 Tyler Street, Port Townsend, WA 98368-6541.

36. Theron G. Randolph, M.D. & Ralph W. Moss, Ph.D., *An Alternative Approach to Allergies*, Bantam Book, July 1982.

37. *The Purification Rundown*, Bridge Publications, Inc., 1414 North Catalina Street, Los Angeles, CA 90027.

38. Royden Brown, *How to Live The Millenium*, Pains Corporation, Phoenix, AZ 85018.

39. Anthony di Fabio, *Germanium*, The Arthritis Trust of America, 7111 Sweetgum Drive SW, Suite A, Fairview, TN 37062-9384.

40. Sandra Goodman, Ph.D., *Germanium, The Health and Life Enhancer*, Thorsons Publishers Limited, Wellingborough, Northamptonshire, NN8 2RQ England.

41. Betty Kamen, Ph.D. *Germanium: A New Approach to Immunity*, Nutrition Encounter, Inc., Box 689, Larkspur, CA 94939.

42. Penny C. Royal, *Herbally Yours*, Sound Nutrition, 2560 North 560 East, Provo, UT 84604, 1987.

43. Yoshide Hagiwara, M.D. *Green Barley Essence*, Keats Publishing Co, 27 Pine St. (Box 876), New Canaan, CT 06840, 1985.

44. Maureen Salaman, *Nutrition: The Cancer Answer*, Stratford Publishing, 1259 El Camino Real, Suite 1500, Menlo Park, CA 94025, 1983.

45. Nathan Pritikin, *The Pritikin Promise*, Pocket

Books, Simon & Schuster, Inc., 1985.

46. Linus Pauling, *How To Live Longer and Feel Better*, Avon Books, 105 Madison Ave., New York, NY 10016, 1986.

47. Anthony di Fabio, *Arthritis*, The Arthritis Trust of America, 7111 Sweetgum Drive SW, Suite A, Fairview, TN 37062-9384

48. Luc De Schepper, M.D., Ph.D., C.A., *Peak Immunity*, 2901 Wilshire Boulevard, Suite 435, Santa Monica, CA 90403, 1989.

49. Dennis W. Remington, M.D., Barbara W. Higa, R.D., *Back to Health*, Vitality House International, Inc., 3707 North Canyon Road #8-C, Provo, UT 84604.

50. Rolf Institute, PO Box 1868, Boulder, CO 80306.

51. Anthony di Fabio, *Chelation Therapy*, The Arthritis Trust of America, 7111 Sweetgum Drive SW, Suite A, Fairview, TN 37062-9384.

52. Anthony di Fabio, *Bee Pollen: The Perfect Food*, The Arthritis Trust of America, 7111 Sweetgum Drive SW, Suite A, Fairview, TN 37062-9384

53. Anthony di Fabio, *The Herxheimer Effect*, The Arthritis Trust of America, 7111 Sweetgum Drive SW, Suite A, Fairview, TN 37062-9384.

54. Robert R. Barefoot, Carl J. Reich, M.D., *The Calcium Factor*, Bokar Consultants, Inc., PO Box 21270, Wickenburg, AZ 85358, 1992.

55. Lida H. Mattman, Ph.D., *Cell Wall Deficient Forms: Stealth Pathogens*, CRC Press, 2000 Corporate Blvd., N.W., Boca Raton, FL 33431, 2nd Edition, 1993.

56. Gerald J. Domingue, Jorgen U. Schlegel, Hannah B. Woody, "Naked Bacteria in Human Blood," *Microbia*, Tome 2, No. 2, Annee 1976.

57. Robert W. Bradford, D.Sc., Henry W. Allen, Michael L. Culbert, D.Sc., *The Biochemical Basis of Live Cell Therapy*," The Robert Bradford Foundation, 1180

Walnut avenue, Chula Vista, California, 92011-2622, May 1986.

The following summarizes everything our foundation has learned about rheumatoid disease since 1982. If you wish to get well, please pay attention!

How Do I Cure

My Rheumatoid Arthritis?

1. How Do I Cure My Rheumatoid Disease?

You start the cure by learning what Rheumatoid Disease is, where it's located in the body, and what causes it. The very first thing to learn is that it is a disease of the whole body, not of your joints. This is true no matter how much your joints ache or how insistent is your friendly neighborhood rheumatologist.

2. Where is Rheumatoid Disease Located in my body?

Rheumatoid Disease is a "systemic" disease. This means that whatever ails you is actually a problem of your whole body — cells, organs, systems — the whole works. If you suffer from Rheumatoid Arthritis, for example, this systemic disease is manifesting itself in your joints. If you suffer from a differently named Rheumatoid Disease, then the target area of your body is given a new name, one different from Rheumatoid Arthritis. In fact, there are about 100 differently named diseases that have essentially the same causes but are known under totally different names as shown at the "Articles" tab, "Arthritis Classifications" at our website http://www.arthritistrust.org.

One of our founders, Professor Roger WyburnMason, M.D., Ph.D., explained this astounding fact by describing the medical profession's past technique for naming tuberculosis before discovery of the tuberculin germ. There were about 100 unique names for apparently different diseases depending upon the part of the body affected. Once the tuberculin bacillus was discovered, all of those names collapsed into TB of the bone, TB of the lung, TB of the skin, and so on.

We think Rheumatoid Disease is a cluster of symptoms named differently — 100 unique names — that can now be understood from the viewpoint of a single, systemic disease. (See "Arthritis Classifications" tab at http:// www.arthritistrust.org.)

3. But what about my immune system? My doctor says that Rheumatoid Arthritis (or Rheumatoid Disease) is caused by a defective immune system?

There may be some folks who have a defective immune system, but these are probably rare. We believe that your immune system is doing exactly what it was constructed to do. By analogy, consider the camel with too many straws on its back. If you remove those straws one or two at a time eventually the camel will be able to stand again. Our recommended treatment protocol does exactly that — removes the stressors from your immune system until your body (and immune system) functions properly again.

Professor Roger Wyburn-Mason again constructed a useful analogy citing past medical history. Prior to the discovery of the syphilis spirochete, the disease of syphilis was often considered a "defective immune system" disease. It displayed all of the characteristics of an immune system gone awry. Once the spirochete was found it was clear to all that this was an infectious disease problem.

Current internal medicine books will often provide two hypotheses for the cause of Rheumatoid Disease: (a) Something is wrong with the immune system, the body is attacking itself; (b) There is one or mor e microorganisms inside the body producing a reaction on the rheumatoid disease victim's tissues, thus causing the manifestation of the disease.

Billions of dollars worth of research following up the "something is wrong with the immune system" has never produced a cure. Whereas tens of thousands — stemming from the 1960s — have gotten well following up on the second, that is that the body is responding to one or more microorganisms.

4. What microorganism causes this terrible disease? Is there only one that affects everyone the same?

When we started the Arthritis Trust of America (The Rheumatoid Disease Foundation) in 1982 we believed that there was but one nasty microorganism, an amoeba. This was according to the findings of Professor Roger Wyburn-Mason and a world-class amoebologist, Dr. Stamm. Dr. Wyburn-Mason was convinced because his treatment designed on the basis of their alleged amoebic findings worked in the large majority of cases. We conducted numerous studies coming at last to the realization that Dr. Wyburn-Mason's treatment protocol was indeed working, but that his belief in an amoebic origin was not necessarily the best answer. (See *The Causation of Rheumatoid Disease and Many Human Cancers*, "Book s and Pamphlets" Ta b, http:// www.arthritistrust.org.)

Meanwhile, independently, Thomas McPherson

Brown, M.D. had concluded that a mycoplasm was the culprit in the creation of Rheumatoid Disease. (See "Thomas McPherso n Brown, M.D. Treatment of Rheumatoid Disease," at "Articles Important" tab of http:// www.arthritistrust.org.)

There are treatments predicated on both of these hypothesis, except that we've added additional, necessary wellness-serving treatment protocols. These are the necessity of correcting nutritional intake, anti-Candidiasis, learn food allergies,clean out root canal infections, get rid of mercury toxification, herbicide and pesticide accumulations, do hormone balancing, and so on.

We now believe that Rheumatoid Disease is caused by many factors (multi-factored) and that there can be one or more out of tens of thousands of invasive microorganisms to which a geneticall y sensitive person's tissues will respond — either to the microorganisms' protein products or to their waste products. This is known as a "genetic susceptibility" to the toxins or protein products of the microorganism.

5. Should I have tests for these microorganisms, these pathogens?

Unless a health professional has some reason to search for a particular pathogen we feel it is a waste of money and time looking for any specific invader by the taking of blood tests or other traditional tests designed to find pathogens. However, Computerized Electrodermal Screening or applied kinesiology are two lowcost, often accurate means for making such a determination, if you wish to make the effort.

Experience has shown, however, that broadspectrum anti-microorganism treatment, coupled with investigation of all the other known causes and assisting treatments, is usually successful, at least 80% of the time.

Here's an example of a patient where our recommended anti-microorganism drugs did not work, but, by following our principles, the patient recovered from

Ankylosing Spondilitis, one of the 100 or so named Rheumatoid Diseases. Reason: he was exposed to a whole different type of invading microorganism than normally found in the United States, *Schistosomiasis bilharzia*, a parasite obtained by swimming in Zimbabwe waters at an altitude where the waters are known to harbor this organism. He was able to get well by using the proper pharmaceutical created for this specific microorganism together with proper application of our other treatment recommendations — that is, unloading the immune system. (See http://www.arthritistrust.org, "Newsletters" "Spring 2005.")

We know patients who achieved wellness using only our recommended anti-microorganism treatments.

We also know of patients who only needed our other recommendations — not the anti-microorganism protocol — and got well.

S o m e patient s requir e m a n y or a l l of our recommendations to achieve wellness.

But, concentrate on the principles we describe and not on a literal-minded authoritarian approach.

6. How will I know exactly what to do? Take the anti-microorganism treatmen t or the other treatments?

Your best bet — if you truly want to get well — is to work with one or more knowledgeable health professionals, and to remove every single suppressor, every straw on the camel's back! You must learn more than your friendly neighborhood rheumatologist. This will be easy to do, because this group of professionals know absolutely nothing about how to get you well (according to their own statements), and you'll know something!

One drawback is this: There's no one health professional or dentist in the United States who offers all the treatment recommendations you will need to explore. Several clinics come close, but the majority of those who originally signed up on our physician referral list were rather limited in what they chose to offer you. So, if you truly want to get well, you should consider several options right at the start.

a. First off, learn everything you can on this website. Especially read the book *Arthritis* by Prosch and di Fabio at http://www.arthritistrust.org, "Books and Pamphlets" tab. Read it end to end.

If you don't understand some of the words, use "Google" or a dictionary or some other search engine to define them. Don't let words stand between you and a good understanding of the principles for achieving wellness. You won't have to learn your friendly neighborhood rheumatologist's complex medical

language, thank goodness, but you'll need to clear up some basic concepts to avoid confusion.

b. After you've learned as much as you feel you can absorb, then start searching for a health professional who will work with you. This could be your family doctor. We'll help her/him to learn, if s/he is openminded and willing to learn.

Otherwise, you can search for a doctor in your geographical region who is dedicated to or inclined to practice alternative/complementary medicine.

Plan on traveling to another location where exists a health professional who will help — and then plan on traveling to another location to visit another health clinic.

To find a biological dentist write or call **The Price-Pottenger Nutrition Foundation**, PO Box

2614, La Mesa, CA 91943-2614; (619) 462-7600.

Or, for a dentist, **American Academy of B i o l o g i c a l   D e n t i s t s** ; h t t p / / www.biologicaldentistry.org

To find a physician for allergies/chemical sensitivities/ addictions **American Academy of Environmental Medicine** call (215) 862-4544)

To find a physician for heart/circulatory problems (chelation therapy) and many other problems write (self-addressed, stamped envelope) **American College for Advancement of Medicine** 23121

Verdugo Dr, Laguna Hills, CA 92653